HOMEOPATHY
MADE SIMPLE

HOMEOPATHY MADE ∼ SIMPLE

A Quick Reference Guide

Dr. R. Donald Papon

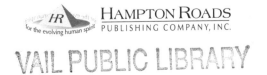

HAMPTON ROADS
PUBLISHING COMPANY, INC.

Cover design by Mayapriya Long
Cover art by John Nguyen

For information write:

Hampton Roads Publishing Company, Inc.
134 Burgess Lane
Charlottesville, VA 22902

Or call: 804-296-2772
FAX: 804-296-5096
e-mail: hrpc@hrpub.com
Web site: http://www.hrpub.com

If you are unable to order this book from your local
bookseller, you may order directly from the publisher.
Quantity discounts for organizations are available.
Call 1-800-766-8009, toll-free.

Library of Congress Catalog Card Number: 98-71592

ISBN 1-57174-110-0

10 9 8 7 6 5 4 3 2 1

Printed on acid-free recycled paper in Canada

This work is dedicated to
Harry Prior . . . journalist . . .
humanitarian . . . whose devotion
to homeopathy serves as an
inspiration for us all!

THE TRUTH ABOUT YOU:
You are what you ARE.
You are what you THINK.
You are what you EAT.
And you are what you DRINK!

GENERAL DISCLOSURE

The conditions for which self-treatment is appropriate are for those symptoms that do not require the immediate care of a physician and do not necessitate complex medical diagnosis or monitoring.

Homeopathy Made Simple is not intended to replace the medical advice of the reader's own healthcare practitioner or to contradict the medical or surgical decisions regarding any ailment of the reader by his or her physician of choice. In no way is the information contained in this book to be considered a prescription for treatment for any disease without the knowledge and consent of the reader's practitioner, who should be personally familiar with the reader's health history.

If your condition worsens or persists, consult your healthcare practitioner.

TABLE OF CONTENTS

II. PROFILES OF THE VARIOUS REMEDIES

Aconitum napellus. Allium cepa. Antimonium tartaricum. Apis mellifica. Arnica montana. Arsenicum album. Belladonna.

Bryonia alba. Calcarea phosphorica. Cantharis. Carbo vegetabilis. Chamomilla. Ferrum phosphoricum. Gelsemium. Hepar sulph. Hypericum perforatum. Ignatia. Ipecac. Ledum palustre. Magnesia phosphorica. Mercurius vivus. Nux vomica. Phosphorus. Pulsatilla. Rhus toxicodendron. Ruta graveolens. Spongia tosta. Sulphur. Veratrum album.

III. FREQUENTLY ASKED QUESTIONS ABOUT HOMEOPATHY

IV. SECRETS OF A PRACTICING HOMEOPATH

FOREWORD

Despite passionately disagreeing with some of the specifics regarding nutritional therapy (I neither use nor recommend any multi-level commissioned—network marketed—products); I can enthusiastically recommend *Homeopathy Made Simple*. Why? Because of its clear usable presentation of homeopathy.

Even though my father was a homeopath early in his career, it was Dr. Don Papon who was directly responsible for my becoming a homeopath. I had, coming from a family with physicians on both sides, resolved to be "not a doctor" until a job in the recreational department of a large state hospital lead me to believe that treating chronic psychiatric illness was my vocation.

A decade later, having been through medical school, an internship, and psychiatric residency, I felt I was further from my goal of finding a better treatment for the mentally unwell than I was while working with my intuition and common sense as a recreational therapist.

I let my discouragement be known and it was suggested that I study with Dr. Carl Pfeiffer, who became my mentor and trained me in nutritional medicine.

While our orthomolecular approach was vastly superior to the heavy drugging used in traditional psychiatry, we had our limitations.

I kept searching for other approaches (meditation, acupuncture, tai chi, etc.), but I always dismissed homeopathy because I thought it was placebo medicine. I believed if it was half as good as my father said, "They threw the baby out with the bath water when they left homeopathy behind; it worked and didn't have the side effects of the drugs we are now using," he would have stayed in general practice instead of specializing in radiology.

One day a patient whom I had referred to Dr. Allan Cott (another founding father in nutritional medicine) returned and let me know that Dr. Cott had said "Bonnet has done everything I can think of. Why don't you see Dr. Papon, a homeopath?" The patient did and improved so dramatically that he had to come back and let me know.

I immediately began studying—reading, going to seminars, etc. Now, over twelve years later, I can say that the study of homeopathy has greatly enhanced my effectiveness as a physician, my personal health, and my development as a human.

Some readers may be blessed enough for *Homeopathy Made Simple* to serve as a catalyst, leading to self-actualization. Most will find it a valuable health manual; it would require a truly closed mind to not be benefited by it.

Philip L. Bonnet, M.D.

INTRODUCTION

How This Work Came to be Written

It is often said that, "Necessity is the mother of invention."

Having practiced and taught homeopathy for over two decades now, I have also come to recognize the great wisdom behind the Master's words, "For many be called, but few chosen."(Matt. 20:16)

While would-be students of homeopathy worldwide have been eager acquirers of a homeopathic household kit (the like of which her Royal Majesty, Queen Elizabeth, never travels without), they have failed to attain that degree of knowledge which is required to make this an essential tool for themselves and their families.

As an educator, however, I know that this is not their fault, as most homoeopathic texts present an air of sophistication far beyond the beginner's needs and comprehension.

While I have long been aware of this chasm in elementary homoeopathic education, it was not until my youngest daughter went away to preparatory school armed with her very own kit that this fact truly struck home.

In the course of the school year, call after call was received with questions as to exactly "which" remedy to take for "what."

While I expect, and actually encourage, such calls from students and clients, this barrage from my very own daughter was much more than I could handle.

In a moment of madness and weakness one day, I promised her I would send her a small guidebook that she could keep by her kit that would answer all such questions and make her truly independent once and for all.

I must say I did this knowing well that one has no need to buy milk if one owns a cow, but somehow the idea of such an addition to the kit began to take shape as a useful tool for anyone, including my precocious daughter.

So, here it is . . . or at least here's the first edition!

This guide, which is really an abbreviated Repertory, has been arranged in the accepted format, except that I have taken out and simplified as much of the medical jargon as possible to make it truly "user friendly."

Problems which are most likely to arise have been placed in **boldface** in order that they may be quickly accessed.

Needless to say, any problem that does not reasonably respond to home care should be directed AT ONCE to one's homeopathic health-care practitioner, whoever he or she may be!

While I sincerely believe that probably 75 percent of all problems encountered in one's daily life can be safely and efficiently dealt with through the use of only 29 remedies, they are not to be thought of as the totality of homeopathic treatment.

On the other hand, as homeopaths, we are often quick to forget that while today we have an army of some 2,000 remedies at our disposal, at the time of Hahnemann's death, only about 99 had been proved.

Hence, homoeopathy must be thought of as a dynamic evolutionary process and not a fixed body of knowledge! Thinking this way allows us to indulge in the fantasy . . . "What if we were shipwrecked on a desert island with only these 29 remedies?"

Surely we would survive and probably even discover other remedies from the local fauna and flora as well! So there you have it in a nutshell.

At the suggestion of the publisher, I have divided this work into four parts. The first part contains a quick, easy way in which to find a remedy that may be useful for a particular problem without the necessity of reading through pages and pages of material.

In part 2, I have outlined the major characteristics of the various remedies contained in the household kit, focusing on the mental aspects of each remedy.

In part 3, I attempt to answer various questions that are often asked when one first encounters homeopathy.

In part 4, I share with you some healthcare secrets I have gleaned from practicing homeopathy for almost two decades in terms of how to treat various underlying causes—which very likely you are not even aware of—but which may be affecting your health adversely!

If you benefit from this guide . . . or have suggestions for future editions . . . please feel free to drop me a line.

Or if you wish . . . just send a "thank you" note to my daughter, who is now in her senior year at college.

Dr. R. Donald Papon
Ocean Grove, New Jersey
Summer 1998

HOW BEST TO
USE THIS BOOK!

In the pages that follow, I have created what homeopaths worldwide call a "Repertory" of the various symptoms you can treat with your own household kit. To find out where such a kit can be obtained, simply refer to the appendix found at the end of this work.

Traditionally, Repertories are arranged in order of the VARIOUS PARTS OF THE BODY, starting with the MIND and its MENTAL SYMPTOMS, and then descending downwards. The parts of the body and their order are as follows:

Mind, Head, Eyes, Nose, Mouth, Face, Stomach, Abdomen, Stool, Urine, Male, Female, Respiratory, Heart, Back, Extremities, Skin, Sleep, Fever, and Modalities, which tell when a person taking a particular remedy feels better or worse.

As an example, right now you have a headache and want to get rid of it! Which remedy should you take? Go to that section marked HEAD (chapter 2) and find that remedy which best describes your condition.

For instance, the headache you have now came from "overwork." First, find the section "Headache" and go down the list until you find the section "overwork." Next to the word "overwork" you will find the abbreviation "PULS." This means that Pulsatilla is the remedy for you to take.

Now let's take another example:

Suppose you have gotten a headache after an encounter with a parent during which you became "angry." Once again go to the section "Headache." If you then go down the list you will find the words "anger, following" which simply means that the headache came *after* you became angry. Next to this you will find the abbreviation "IGN," which means that "Ignatia" is the remedy for you to take.

If more than one remedy is indicated for a particular problem, you can either start with one remedy and give it some time to work, or you can alternate between the various remedies, taking one and another a few hours later.

How often should you take this remedy? If the condition you are treating is ACUTE, you may take this remedy every 1-2 hours or even every half hour if necessary. If the condition is CHRONIC, however, taking the remedy twice or three times daily will suffice. If you are treating a CHRONIC condition, it will take some time for you to correct this condition.

It is a generally accepted rule of homeopathic healing that it takes "one month of treatment for every year a person has been ill" in order to recover.

This means then, if you have had a health problem of three years standing, it is unrealistic for you to expect to get completely well in just a few WEEKS of treatment!

Ill for three years? Give yourself "three months" to get well!

Those conditions that have been found to occur very frequently I have placed in **boldface** type so you can find them more quickly.

One final comment. If you do NOT find relief from a particular problem after a reasonable time of self-treatment, consult your healthcare practitioner.

I

YOUR
FIVE-MINUTE
PRESCRIBER

REMEDIES INCLUDED IN YOUR HOMEOPATHIC KIT*

Latin Name	Common Name	Abbreviation
Aconitum napellus	Monkshood	ACON
Allium cepa	Red Onion	ALL-C
Antimonium tartaricum	Potash	ANT-T
Apis mellifica	Honey Bee	APIS
Arnica montana	Leopard's Bane	ARN
Arsenicum album	Arsenic Oxide	ARS
Belladonna	Deadly Nightshade	BELL
Bryonia alba	Wild Hops	BRY
Calcarea phosphorica	Calcium Phosphate	CALC-P
Cantharis	Spanish Fly	CANTH
Carbo vegetabilis	Vegetable Charcoal	CARB-V
Chamomilla	German Chamomile	CHAM
Ferrum phosphoricum	Phosphate of Iron	FER-P
Gelsemium	Yellow Jasmine	GELS

Latin Name	Common Name	Abbreviation
Hepar sulph	Calcium Sulphide	HEP
Hypericum perforatum	St. John's Wort	HYPER
Ignatia	St. Ignatius Bean	IGN
Ipecac	Ipecac Root	IP
Ledum palustre	Marsh Tea	LED
Magnesia phosphorica	Magnesium Phosphate	MAG-P
Mercurius vivus	Mercury	MERC
Nux vomica	Poison Nut	NUX
Phosphorus	Phosphorus	PHOS
Pulsatilla	Wind Flower	PULS
Rhus toxicodendron	Poison Ivy	RHUS
Ruta graveolens	Rue Bitterwort	RUTA
Spongia tosta	Roasted Sponge	SPONG
Sulphur	Sulphur	SULPH
Veratrum album	White Hellebore	VERAT-A

*These are the remedies that commonly appear in most homeopathic household kits. Readers wishing to obtain a kit for themselves are referred to the appendix of this work for various sources.

CHAPTER I

MIND Your Own Business

Keep the following conditions and remedies "in mind" as you seek specific remedies in the chapters that follow. Early homeopaths referred to the "three-legged stool" process of choosing a remedy. Considering your state of mind is the third "leg," but first:

As instructed earlier, go to the chapter for a condition in a particular part of the body, use the remedy suggested there, and wait for it to work. If for some reason you cannot figure out which remedy, or you are torn between two different remedies, then consult with this section and take which remedy matches your mental state. You can also consult this section if you take a remedy that should be correct but you do not get any results after using it for a reasonable amount of time. The MIND section should be used only if you cannot arrive at a remedy by other means.

MIND	
Affectionate	PULS
Alone, wants to be	GELS
"	ARN

MIND	
Anger	**BRY**
esp. with menses	**CHAM**
,,	**HEP**
,,	**NUX**
Anxiety	ACON
,,	ARS
,,	CALC-P
,,	SPONG
Apathy	APIS
Brooding	IGN
Depression	**ARS**
,,	**GELS**
,,	**SULPH**
before menses	**PHOS**
after injury	**HYPER**
Despair	ARS
,,	IGN
Despondency	ANT-T
Disappointment	IGN
Dissatisfied	BRY
Emotional	GELS
,,	PULS
Faultfinding	NUX
Fear	
agoraphobia	ARN
being alone	ANT-T
crowds	**ACON**
darkness	CARB-V
death	ACON
,,	ARS
,,	PHOS
disaster	SULPH
ghosts	CARB-V
heights	HYPER

MIND	
immobilized by	ACON
losing mind	MERC
seasickness	**ACON**
stage fright	**GELS**
touch	ARN
thunder	PHOS
Fickle	PULS
Fidgety	PHOS
Forgetful,	CALC-P
very	SULPH
Fretful	NUX
infants	CHAM
at menses	CHAM
Furious	BELL
Gentle	PULS
Gloomy	PHOS
Grief	IGN
,,	APIS
Hallucination	BELL
Hopeless	ARS
,,	IGN
Impatient	BRY
,,	CHAM
Indifferent	ARS
,,	FER-P
,,	PHOS
,,	VERAT-A
Intellectual	NUX
Intense	BRY
,,	NUX
Insane	FER-P
Introspective	IGN
Irritable	ARS
,,	BRY

MIND	
,,	CHAM
slight cause	HEP
everything	IP
,,	NUX
,,	SULPH
Jealousy	APIS
Laughing, easily	PULS
Lazy	SULPH
Listless	GELS
Mania, acute	CANTH
Melancholy	HYPER
,,	IGN
religious	SULPH
with stupor	VERAT-A
Memory	
loss	**PHOS**
poor	**CARB-V**
weak	**MERC**
Mild	PULS
Miserly	ARS
Morose	ARN
Pain	
attacks of	SULPH
complaints of	MAG-P
Peevish	CHAM
People, aversion to	CHAM
Quarrelsome	NUX
Questions, slow to answer	MERC
Rage	APIS
,,	CANTH
Restless	ACON
,,	ARS
,,	BELL
,,	CHAM

MIND	
,,	SULPH
after midnight	ARS
anxious with	CANTH
emotional with	ACON
extreme	ARS
physical	ACON
,,	SULPH
whining with	CHAM
Sadness	HEP
,,	IGN
Selfish,	ARS
extremely	SULPH
Sensitive,	PHOS
extremely	HEP
Sensitive to:	
alcohol	NUX
coffee	NUX
criticism	NUX
everything	NUX
,,	PHOS
lights	NUX
,,	PHOS
mental exertion	NUX
music	NUX
noise	NUX
,,	PHOS
odors	NUX
,,	PHOS
other people	NUX
spices	NUX
tobacco smoke	NUX
touch	NUX
,,	PHOS
slightly sensitive to those above	HEP

MIND	
Shock, after	HYPER
„	IGN
Shrieks	VERAT-A
Sighing	IGN
Slow comprehension	CALC-P
Stupid, feels	ACON
appears	VERAT-A
Suicidal,	ARS
at night	HEP
Sullen	VERAT-A
Thinking	
poor	**NUX**
slow	**CARB-V**
unclear	**MAG-P**
Thoughts, vanish	NUX
Thunderstorms, fear of	PHOS
Travels constantly	CALC-P
Unhappiness	ACON
Weary of life	PHOS
Weeping	BELL
„	PULS
Whining	APIS
Will power, loss of	MERC
Withdrawn, from life	PHOS
Work	
aversion to	SULPH
complains about	HEP
confused as to	GELS
curses at	VERAT-A
lacks courage for	ARS
mood changes at	BELL
„	IGN
poor concentration at	APIS
shows conceit	PHOS

MIND	
shows contempt for	IP
talks excessively of	BRY
Workaholic	SULPH
Worry	ACON
Writing, mistakes in	HYPER

CHAPTER 2

It's All in the HEAD!

HEAD	
Alive, feels	HYPER
Bones, brittle	
in children	CALC-P
feel crushed	IP
Brain fatigue	HYPER
,,	PHOS
Cap on head, feels as if	MAG-P
Cold feeling	CALC-P
Dizziness	GELS
in aged	CALC-P
,,	PHOS
chronic	ARN
confusion with	ANT-T
consciousness, loss of	NUX
dinner, after	NUX
lying on back	MERC
morning	NUX
moving while	MAG-P
open air	CANTH
riding, while	HEP
rising, on	ACON
,,	BRY

HEAD	
"	RHUS
shaking head	HEP
sneezing with	APIS
stooping, worse	SULPH
walking, when	ARN
"	LED
Fontanelles, unclosed	CALC-P
Forehead	
hot	BELL
"	SULPH
cold	VERAT-A
Hair	
splits	BELL
falls out	CARB-V
"	HYPER
"	MERC
"	PHOS
"	SULPH
Headache	**BELL**
air, improves	ALL-C
worsens	NUX
alcohol, after	NUX
"	RUTA
anger, following	IGN
band around head, feels like	GELS
"	ANT-T
"	MERC
blindness, before	GELS
burning	ACON
bursting	SPONG
catarrhal	ALL-C
children, esp. at puberty	CALC-P
close room	HYPER
coffee, after	NUX

HEAD	
cold improves	FER-P
cold sweat	HEP
confusion with	ARN
congestive	FER-P
during menses	GELS
eyes	BELL
"	BRY
"	HYPER
"	MERC
"	RHUS
face, extends to	PULS
forehead	ALL-C
"	BELL
"	SPONG
with cold spot	ARN
fullness	ACON
grief, following	IGN
hair cut, after	BELL
hemorrhoids with	NUX
light worsens	BELL
lying down worsens	BELL
mental labor	MAG-P
motion worsens	BRY
nail, feels like	IGN
"	NUX
"	RUTA
noise worsens	BELL
"	FER-P
overwork	PULS
periodic	SULPH
pressing outward	ACON
pressure, improves	APIS
pulsating,	BELL
right side	BELL

HEAD	
root of nose	IGN
sharp, pinching	ARN
sinus	BRY
spinal injury	HYPER
splitting	BRY
stabbing, sudden	APIS
sun, ill effects	FER-P
,,	NUX
teeth, pain extends to	IP
,,	PULS
temples	BELL
throbbing	FER-P
,,	APIS
one half head	CHAM
vertex	HYPER
tobacco, worsens	IGN
,,	NUX
top, heat on	SULPH
touch, sensitive to	BELL
urination, improves	GELS
warm room	ALL-C
weather, change in	CALC-P
hollow, feels	IGN
liquid, as if	MAG-P
longer, feels	HYPER
scalp itches	CANTH
,,	HEP
soreness, to touch	FER-P
sweating	CALC-P
top of, warm	ACON

CHAPTER 3

The EYES Have It!

EYES	
Adjusting for distance, spasm when	IP
Alcohol, irritates	NUX
Black	
bruised	**RUTA**
tender, swollen	**LED**
trauma	**APN**
Blue circles	
around	ARS
under	PHOS
Blurred vision	MAG-P
Bruising to	LED
Burning	ALL-C
"	CANTH
Cataract	PHOS
Close work worsens	ARN
"	IP
Circles, sees	HEP
Colored lights, sees	MAG-P
Conjunctivitis	
early stages	**ACON**
acute	**APIS**
burning	ARS

EYES	
dilation, pupils	BELL
hot feeling	SULPH
rubbing eyes	PULS
sand, feels like	FER-P
shingles	RHUS
weeping	PULS
Cornea, ulcer	ARS
„	HEP
„	SULPH
opacity	CALC-P
Discharge	
irritating	ALL-C
mucus	SPONG
running	ALL-C
„	PULS
Discoloration, from injury	LED
Dizzy, on closing	ARN
Eyeball sore	FER-P
Eyeglasses, helps	GELS
Floaters, black	CARB-V
„	MERC
„	PHOS
„	SULPH
Foreign body, in	ARN
„	HYPER
„	LED
Glass, feels like in eye	SULPH
Glaucoma	
acute	ACON
„	BELL
double vision	GELS
elderly	PHOS
intraocular, tension	BRY
painful	PHOS

EYES	
Hemorrhage, retinal	ARN
Illusions	BELL
Inflammation	ACON
”	SULPH
after injury	ARN
cold worsens	RHUS
damp worsens	RHUS
in newborn	ACON
”	SULPH
Letters, appear red	PHOS
Lids	
burning	ALL-C
close, spasmatic	CHAM
dry	VERAT-A
red	MERC
swollen	APIS
”	RHUS
Light, irritates	ALL-C
”	ARS
”	NUX
”	RHUS
Television, watching	ARN
Moving, sore when	BRY
Pain	
muscles	CARB-V
neuralgia	IGN
piercing	APIS
Pupils, contracted	MAG-P
dilated	BELL
Reading, vision worsened by	HEP
Redness of	ACON
”	FER-P
Retina, detatched	GELS
Rings, around	VERAT-A

EYES	
Sand, feels like	FER-P
Sensitivity,	ACON
light	BELL
sight, when straining to see	ARN
Strain	
aches	**LED**
double vision	**GELS**
overwork	**RUTA**
Styes	APIS
"	PULS
"	SULPH
Swelling	
around	ARS
protruding	BELL
underneath	APIS
Tearing	ACON
"	ALL-C
profuse	IP
Tired	ARN
Throbbing	BELL
Tobacco, irritates	NUX
Touch, sore to	BRY
"	HEP
Warm room, irritates	PULS
Watering	BELL
"	SPONG
Weakness, upper eyelids	GELS
Wounds, contusion	LED
Zigzags, sees	IGN

CHAPTER 4

Can You EAR
What I Am Saying?

EARS	
Aching around	CALC-P
Bleeding from	ARN
"	RHUS
Boils	MERC
Coldness	VERAT
Dryness	CARB-V
Earache, acute	**ACON**
cold air/water	MAG-P
crying because of	BELL
discharge with	HEP
"	MERC
"	RHUS
"	SULPH
fever with	ACON
"	MERC
first sign of	FER-P
getting wet	PULS
headache with	BELL
itchiness with	SULPH

EARS	
left ear	HEP
noise bothers	NUX
recurring	SULPH
right ear	BELL
,,	MAG-P
sharp pain	MERC
sore throat with	BELL
,,	HEP
shooting (radiating)	ALL-C
swelling	APIS
throbbing	BELL
unbearable	CHAM
wind or draft	HEP
Eustachian tube	ALL-C
,,	BELL
Glands below, swollen	ARN
,,	BELL
Hearing	
acute	BELL
echo in	PHOS
lost	ARN
,,	FER-P
Hot air, feeling	CANTH
Illness, after	CARB-V
Inflamed	APIS
,,	PULS
,,	SULPH
Itching	NUX
Music unbearable	ACON
Noise	
in	ARN
,,	FER-P
bothers	ACON
buzzing	BRY

EARS	
ringing	CHAM
roaring	ARS
"	BRY
whizzing	SULPH
Odor from	PULS
Stopped, feeling	CHAM
Stuffed, feeling	PULS
Voice, hard to hear	PHOS
Water, feels like in left ear	ACON
Wind, feeling	CANTH

CHAPTER 5

I NOSE What You're Doing!

NOSE	
Acne	ARS
Bleeding	**FER-P**
red blood	ACON
"	ARN
"	BELL
handkerchief, on, after blowing nose	PHOS
menses, during	BRY
morning	NUX
nighttime	MERC
stooping, while	RHUS
Bones swollen	MERC
sore	PULS
Catarrh, chronic	PULS
"	SULPH
Common Cold	
bleeding	FER-P
burning discharge	ARS
chills	GELS
cold air worsens	BRY
disposed to	CALC-P

NOSE	
"	FER-P
early stage	ACON
"	FER-P
headache with	NUX
intolerable	NUX
later stages	HEP
nausea	IP
open air improves	PULS
rapid onset	GELS
shiver & chills	GELS
sleep, cannot	CHAM
sneezing	ALL-C
"	MERC
sore throat with	MERC
watery discharge	ALL-C
Damp weather, worsened by	MERC
Discharge	ALL-C
acrid	ALL-C
bland	ALL-C
burning	ALL-C
colored	PULS
green	MERC
irritating	ALL-C
morning, in	PULS
profuse	ALL-C
"	MERC
running	ACON
thick	PULS
watery	ALL-C
"	MERC
Dry inside	ACON
"	GELS
"	SPONG
"	SULPH

NOSE	
Hay Fever	
dry sneezing	**ARS**
fall worsens	**ALL-C**
open air improves	**PULS**
spring worsens	**ALL-C**
Herpes, across	SULPH
Inflamed	APIS
,,	RHUS
Odors, imagines	BELL
,,	PHOS
,,	SULPH
Open air worsens	ARS
,,	NUX
Pain on touch	RHUS
Polyps nasal	ALL-C
,,	SULPH
bleed easily	PHOS
catarrh excess	PULS
Red	APIS
,,	BELL
,,	RHUS
Sinusitis	
hypersensitive	HEP
pain in front	BELL
pain above eyes	PULS
Smell	
catarrh yellow	HEP
lost sense of	PULS
open air improves	PULS
sensitivity of	CHAM
Sneezing	**ALL-C**
,,	**GELS**
without relief	**ARS**
unable to stop	**CARB-V**

NOSE	
Soreness	MERC
feels as if	ARN
nostrils	CALC-P
Stopped up	ACON
"	IP
alternate sides	NUX
indoors	SULPH
night, at	NUX
right nostril	PULS
Throbbing	ACON
Tip of	
cold	APIS
red	RHUIS
scabby	CARB-V
swollen	BRY
tingles	BELL
Varicose veins on	CARB-V
Warm room worsens	ALL-C

CHAPTER 6

FACE It . . .
This Stuff Works!

FACE	
Aches	FER-P
Acne	**HEP**
"	**SULPH**
Blue	ANT-T
"	VERAT-A
Blue rings, eyes	IP
"	PHOS
Bluish-Red	BELL
Cheeks	
bites inside	IGN
red pimples	LED
sore	FER-P
sunken	ARS
tearing	VERAT-A
tingling	ACON
mottled	CARB-V
one red, one pale	CHAM
Chin, quivers	ANT-T
"	GELS
Cold	ANT-T

FACE	
icy, esp. nose	VERAT-A
with cold sweat	CARB-V
Collapsed	VERAT-A
Color changes	IGN
Contracted	GELS
Death-like	CANTH
Dirty looking	MERC
Earthy	MERC
Eruption	
crusty	LED
"	RHUS
eyebrows	SULPH
red patches	ACON
"	ARN
Flushed	ACON
"	FER-P
"	GELS
Greasy	CALC-P
Hot	ACON
"	BELL
with urinary symptoms	CANTH
"	FER-P
"	GELS
Itching, vesicles	CANTH
Jaws, crack	RHUS
dislocate	RHUS
Jerking muscles	CHAM
Lips	
black	BRY
bright red	SULPH
cracked,	**BRY**
"	**HEP**
in the middle	PULS
dry	BRY

FACE	
frequently licks	PULS
swollen	APIS
Lower jaw dropped	GELS
Neuralgia	ACON
"	FER-P
esp. right side	HEP
Numbness	ACON
Pain, jaws	ACON
opening, when	CALC-P
piercing	APIS
shooting	HEP
Pale	ARS
"	ANT-T
"	APIS
"	CANTH
"	CARB-V
"	IP
"	PHOS
very	VERAT-A
Perspiring	CARB-V
cold sweat	ANT-T
Pinched	CARB-V
Puffy	CARB-V
"	MERC
Red	ACON
"	APIS
"	BELL
"	CHAM
"	FER-P
"	SULPH
alternate with pale	ACON
pimples, forehead	LED
Shiny	BELL
Sickly	PHOS

FACE	
Sunken	VERAT-A
Swollen	ACON
,,	APIS
,,	RHUS
lower jaw especially	PHOS
upper lip especially	BELL
,,	CHAM
Twitching	BELL
face & lips	IGN
Waxy	APIS
Wizened	PHOS
Yellowish	HEP

CHAPTER 7

Close Yo' MOUTH!

MOUTH, GUMS & TONGUE	
Breath	
fetid	ARN
horrible	MERC
offensive	PULS
Burned by food	CANTH
Gums	
bleed easily	ARS
"	HEP
"	PHOS
when cleaning	CARB-V
hot inflamed	ACON
spongy	MERC
swollen	APIS
"	SULPH
Mouth	
burning	CANTH
cool sensation	VERAT-A
dry	ACON
"	BELL
"	BRY
"	VERAT-A
edges dry	RHUS

MOUTH, GUMS & TONGUE	
glossy	APIS
"	PULS
numb	ACON
painful	HEP
shiny	APIS
thirsty	ARN
"	BRY
"	MERC
ulcers	ARS
"	MERC
salivation, extra	MERC
at night	CHAM
twitching	MAG-P
Saliva	
bloody	ARS
"	NUX
salty	VERAT-A
sweet	PULS
Taste	
bitter	ARN
"	BRY
"	NUX
"	SULPH
changes	PULS
foul	PULS
greasy	PULS
metallic	ARS
musty	LED
putrid	GELS
rotten eggs	ARN
sour	IGN
"	NUX
sweet	MERC
Thrush, candida	**CANTH**

MOUTH, GUMS & TONGUE

,,	**CARB-V**
,,	**NUX**
Tongue	
clean, red	ARS
half furry	NUX
coated brown	ANT-T
,,	BRY
,,	NUX
white	ACON
cracked	BRY
dry	BRY
dry & brown	SPONG
edges cracked	NUX
fiery red	APIS
furrow, upper	MERC
furry	CANTH
moist & white	PULS
numb	CALC-P
painful	BELL
paralyzed	GELS
pasty	ANT-T
raw	APIS
red	ARS
red & dry center	ANT-T
red edges	BELL
scalded	APIS
strawberry	BELL
swollen	ACON
,,	BELL
teeth indented	MERC
thick, white	ANT-T
tip, red	NUX
,,	SULPH
red triangle	RHUS

MOUTH, GUMS & TONGUE	
tingles	ACON
vesicles, full	SPONG
white	BRY
“	NUX
yellowish	BRY
“	MERC
yellow-brown	CARB-V

CHAPTER 8

SMILE . . . You're on Candid Camera!

TEETH	
Abscess	APIS
Anesthesia, after	**CHAM**
Chewing painful	MERC
Coffee, worse from	CHAM
”	IGN
Cold, sensitive to	ACON
”	NUX
Cold, improves	PULS
Decay	CALC-P
especially crowns	MERC
Dry socket	RUTA
Extraction, bleeds	PHOS
Fear of work on	ACON
”	GELS
Grinding of	BELL
Heavy, feel	VERAT-A
Hot foods, better	MAG-P
Loose	MERC
”	RHUS
Neuralgia, burning	ARS

TEETH	
Night, worse	CHAM
Pain	
intolerable	**CHAM**
shooting	**BELL**
throbbing	**BELL**
to reduce	**HYPER**
Pregnancy, worse	CHAM
Sensitive, chewing	CARB-V
Smoking, worse	IGN
Surgery	
before	**ARN**
after	**ARN**
"	**HYPER**
"	**RUTA**
Teething	ACON
"	CHAM
complicated	CALC-P
"	CHAM
convulsions with	MAG-P
delayed	MAG-P
tender, feels	MERC
too long, feels	MERC
"	RHUS
Toothache	**MERC**
"	**NUX**
when hand-washing clothes	PHOS
"	VERAT-A
Touching painful	MERC
Warm food, worse	CHAM

CHAPTER 9

No Draculas Allowed!

THROAT	
Aching all over	MAG-P
Adenoid, growths	CALC-P
Burned, after hot food	CANTH
Burning	**ACON**
,,	ARS
,,	CANTH
,,	GELS
,,	MERC
,,	SPONG
,,	SULPH
Choking,	MAG-P
tendency to	IGN
Constricted	ACON
,,	APIS
,,	MAG-P
,,	ARS
feels like	BELL
,,	BRY
Dryness	ACON
,,	BELL
,,	SULPH
,,	BRY

THROAT	
great	SPONG
Eating, better by solid food	IGN
Fire, feels like	CANTH
Fishbone, feels like	APIS
Glazed, appears	BELL
Hair, feels like	SULPH
Hoarseness,	ALL-C
,,	ANT-T
,,	BELL
,,	CHAM
,,	HEP
,,	SPONG
with cough	MERC
from overuse	ARN
,,	CALC-P
,,	CARB-V
,,	PHOS
painless	BELL
worse in evening	PHOS
Laryngitis	**FER-P**
Liquids, worsen	BELL
Lump in, feels like	GELS
,,	IGN
Mucus in	BRY
Night, worse at	BELL
,,	CARB-V
Pain goes to ear	GELS
Parotid glands, swollen	CHAM
Red,	**ACON**
especially right side	**BELL**
,,	**MAG-P**
Scalded, feels	CANTH
Scraped, feels	BELL
,,	BRY

THROAT	
,,	NUX
Singing worsens	FER-P
Soreness, right side	**MAG-P**
,,	**MERC**
Spasms	BELL
Splinter, like	HEP
,,	SULPH
Stiffness, right side	MAG-P
Stinging	ACON
,,	APIS
Stitches to ear	IGN
,,	NUX
Surgery, after	FER-P
Swallow	
cannot	ARS
constant desire	MERC
difficult	GELS
ear pain	GELS
sticking	BRY
Swollen,	
inside & out	APIS
,,	ARS
bluish-red	MERC
talking, worse by	CARB-V
Thyroid gland, swollen	SPONG
Tickling	ALL-C
,,	ARN
,,	LED
,,	NUX
Tonsils	
dry	ACON
enlarged	BELL
fiery red	APIS
inflamed	IGN

THROAT	
puffy	APIS
swollen	ACON
,,	CALC-P
,,	APIS
,,	FER-P
,,	IGN
ulcers	APIS
,,	IGN
Uvula, swollen	APIS
,,	NUX
Voice lost	**BELL**
,,	**HEP**
completely	MERC
weak	VERAT-A
Warm food, worsens	GELS
Warm room, worsens	BRY
Wind, dry cold, worsens	HEP

CHAPTER 10

One Man's Poison!

DIGESTION	
Abdomen distended	CARB-V
"	CHAM
"	HEP
"	MERC
"	PULS
"	RHUS
Acids, sensitivity to	MAG-P
All-gone feeling	IGN
"	PULS
Amebic dysentery	IP
Anxiety in pit of	ARS
Appetite, excess	SULPH
Appetite, loss of	ACON
"	BELL
"	CALC-P
"	RHUS
complete loss of	SULPH
Aversion to	
butter	PULS
fats	CARB-V
"	HEP
"	PULS

DIGESTION	
meat	BELL
,,	CARB-V
,,	FER-P
milk	BELL
,,	CARB-V
,,	FER-P
warm food	PULS
Belching	**ALL-C**
difficult	**NUX**
much wind	**PHOS**
with no relief	**MAG-P**
Bloating, after eating	NUX
Body rigid	IP
Burning	ACON
,,	HEP
with thirst	CANTH
Clothing,	
must loosen	MAG-P
,,	PULS
,,	SPONG
Cold water, improved by	ACON
thirst for	ANT-T
Cramps	IGN
Cutting pains	IP
Desire for	
acids	ARS
,,	HEP
,,	IGN
apples	ANT-T
bacon	CALC-P
coffee	ARS
cold drinks	CHAM
,,	MERC
,,	PHOS

DIGESTION	
,,	SULPH
cold foods	PHOS
dirt	MERC
fats	NUX
fruits	ANT-T
ham	CALC-P
indigestible foods	IGN
milk	APIS
,,	ARS
,,	RHUS
salted food	CALC-P
,,	CARB-V
,,	PHOS
spices	HEP
,,	NUX
,,	SULPH
stimulants	FER-P
sugar	MAG-P
sweets	SULPH
vinegar	ARN
wine	HEP
,,	HYPER
Digestion, slow	CARB-V
weak	MERC
Disgust, for everything	CANTH
Dizziness, after eating	RHUS
Drinking, dread of	BELL
Eructations,	
burning	MAG-P
gaseous	CALC-P
Flatulence	**CALC-P**
,,	**PULS**
much	**IGN**
Gastralgia	MAG-P

DIGESTION	
"	RUTA
Gastritis	FER-P
Gnawing, hungry	PULS
Heartburn	CALC-P
"	PULS
Heavy load, feels like	GELS
Hiccough	**IP**
"	**MAG-P**
"	**MERC**
evening	**GELS**
spasmodic	**BELL**
"	**VERAT-A**
Hunger	
after eating	PHOS
continuous	MERC
great	SPONG
ravenous	NUX
"	ALL-C
Indigestion	
acids	ARS
coffee	CANTH
"	CHAM
"	NUX
half hour after eating	CARB-V
hour after eating	PULS
ice cream	ARS
milk	SULPH
summer heat	BRY
tobacco, use of	ARS
vinegar	ARS
Liver, enlarged	MERC
"	NUX
pain in	SULPH
Lump, feels like a	HYPER

DIGESTION	
Melons, ill effect	ARS
Nausea	**ALL-C**
,,	FER-P
,,	IP
,,	PULS
after eating	ANT-T
,,	NUX
,,	RHUS
and vomiting	MAG-P
,,	NUX
constant	IP
fear, causes	ANT-T
morning	CARB-V
,,	NUX
when rising	BRY
Navel, worse near	IP
Pain, after food	CALC-P
bending double	MAG-P
cold food, better	PHOS
right side	RHUS
stabbing	MERC
Pressure in stomach	BRY
Regurgitation	MAG-P
Retching, empty	BELL
day & night	MAG-P
Salt, bad effects	PHOS
Sinking feeling	IGN
Taste remains after eating	PULS
Thirst	
after drinking cold water	BELL
,,	MAG-P
,,	VERAT-A
great	ARS
intense	ACON

DIGESTION	
"	MERC
none	APIS
"	GELS
"	PULS
unquenchable	CANTH
"	RHUS
Sight of food, cannot bear	ARS
Simplest food distresses	CARB-V
Sleepy after eating	RHUS
Smell of food, cannot bear	ARS
Spasms	BELL
Sweat, with profuse	ACON
after eating	CHAM
Urination, with	ACON
Vegetables, ill effects	ARS
Vomiting	
after cold water	CALC-P
after eating	ARS
"	BRY
after anything	VERAT-A
alternating with diarrhea	VERAT-A
before breakfast	FER-P
better after	NUX
bitter	CHAM
blood	ARN
"	FER-P
fear causes	ACON
food	APIS
"	IP
infantile	CALC-P
post-operative	PHOS
right side, except when lying on	ANT-T
sweat, profuse	ACON
uncontrollable	BELL

DIGESTION

undigested food	FER-P
Walking, worsens	PHOS
Water, feeling filled up after drinking	SULPH
Weak at 11 a.m.	SULPH

CHAPTER II

What Goes in Comes Out!

RECTUM & STOOL	
Anus	
blood discharged	CARB-V
burning	CARB-V
"	SULPH
fistula	CALC-P
"	LED
start of	RHUS
heat	ALL-C
itching	ACON
"	CARB-V
"	IGN
"	SULPH
paralyzed	GELS
pain	ACON
pressure in	ARS
prolapsus	RUTA
"	SULPH
redness	SULPH
skin torn	ARS
stitches	ALL-C

RECTUM & STOOL	
"	IGN
uneasiness	NUX
Colic, infantile	CALC-P
Constipation	
"	**IGN**
"	**NUX**
"	**SULPH**
cold drinks worsen	BRY
diarrhea,	BRY
alternating with	NUX
desire for stool absent	BRY
elderly, in the	**CALC-P**
frequent, but no success	SULPH
hot weather, worse	BRY
inactivity, rectum	VERAT-A
infantile	MAG-P
painful stool	SULPH
Diarrhea	
"	**CHAM**
"	**PHOS**
after cold drink	ACON
"	BRY
"	PULS
in hot weather	ARS
blood streaked	IP
chronic	SULPH
cold weather	IP
"	MERC
"	NUX
constipation, alternates with	NUX
drinking, after	ARS
eating, after	APIS
"	ARS
elderly, in the	CARB-V

RECTUM & STOOL	
emotional cause	GELS
fright, from	GELS
,,	IGN
fruit, from	CALC-P
menses, before	VERAT-A
morning	SULPH
night, worse	ARS
pain, burning	ARN
painless	ARS
,,	SULPH
profuse with vomiting	VERAT-A
protracted	SULPH
reddish mucus	RHUS
slimy	NUX
slimy green	CHAM
smelly	CHAM
strange food	IP
teething	MERC
,,	SULPH
vomiting with	IP
,,	VERAT-A
warm weather	BRY
watery	MAG-P
Dysentery	**FER-P**
,,	**CANTH**
,,	**PULS**
,,	**RHUS**
Gallstones	CALC-P
colic	MAG-P
Hemorrhoids	
,,	**FER-P**
,,	**NUX**
,,	**SULPH**
backache with	BELL

RECTUM & STOOL	
bathing worsens	SULPH
improves	NUX
bleeding	HYPER
,,	PHOS
blind	PULS
bluish	CARB-V
burning	ARS
,,	CARB-V
,,	SULPH
cold air, improves	SULPH
confinement, after	APIS
constipation, from	NUX
coughing worsens	IGN
heat, improves	ARS
itching	NUX
,,	SULPH
painful	CHAM
,,	HYPER
recurrent	SULPH
standing, worse	SULPH
stinging pain	APIS
Stool	
dark	APIS
,,	BRY
dry	BRY
,,	SULPH
as if burnt	BRY
,,	SULPH
alcohol, worsened by	ARS
bleeding, after	CALC-P
bloody	APIS
,,	ARN
,,	CANTH
burning follows	CARB-V

RECTUM & STOOL	
cadaverous smell	CARB-V
,,	RHUS
clay colored	HEP
cream colored	GELS
cutting colic	MERC
dog's, like	PHOS
expel, cannot	HEP
,,	PHOS
,,	RUTA
foul smelling	ALL-C
,,	ARN
,,	SULPH
frequent	ARN
,,	CARB-V
frothy	RHUS
green	BELL
,,	CHAM
,,	MERC
hard	PHOS
,,	SULPH
involuntary	APIS
,,	PHOS
knotty	SULPH
large	BRY
,,	SULPH
,,	VERAT-A
lie down after, must	ARN
long, narrow	PHOS
lumps, chalklike	BELL
meat, spoiled	ARS
morning, worse	BRY
moving, worse	BRY
never-get-done, feeling	MERC
night, worse at	ARS

RECTUM & STOOL

no two alike	PULS
odor of rotten eggs	CHAM
painful	SULPH
„	BELL
putrid	IP
scanty	NUX
shivering with	CANTH
slimy	ARN
small, frequent	ACON
offensive	ARS
sour odor	MERC
stinging	BELL
thin	BELL
undigested food	FER-P
„	HEP
urination with	APIS
watery	CHAM
„	FER-P
„	MERC
weakness, after	PHOS
white-grey	MERC
white-yellow mucous	CHAM
worms, thread	FER-P

CHAPTER 12

Please Don't
Wet the Daisies!

URINARY	
Acute infections	BELL
Bladder	
burning in	ACON
elderly, of	HEP
full, feels	RUTA
irritable	NUX
irritation	FER-P
paralyzed	ARS
"	GELS
stone in	CALC-P
weakness	ALL-C
Blowing the nose, kidney pain when	CALC-P
Lifting, kidney pain when	CALC-P
Orchitis	ANT-T
Urethra	
burning in	ACON
"	ALL-C
"	ANT-T
"	CANTH
"	PULS

URINARY	
"	SULPH
discharge from	MERC
itching in	NUX
weakness	ALL-C
Urination	
bedwetting	SULPH
burning	**APIS**
"	**ARS**
"	**CANTH**
copious	CALC-P
"	SULPH
constant	RUTA
continuous	BELL
cough, with	FER-P
"	PULS
"	VERAT-A
cutting	CANTH
diabetes	ARS
"	FER-P
dribbling	NUX
drop by drop	CANTH
excess	FER-P
frequent	APIS
"	BELL
"	MERC
"	NUX
"	RHUS
"	SULPH
incontinence	APIS
"	BELL
"	CALC-P
"	FER-P
increased	ANT-T
"	CALC-P

URINARY	
intolerable, urging	CANTH
involuntary	ARS
irritation	APIS
last drop, burns	APIS
little	NUX
lying down	PULS
must hurry	SULPH
nighttime	PULS
”	SULPH
painful	ACON
”	CANTH
”	RHUS
pregnancy, in	BELL
”	NUX
”	PULS
profuse	ACON
”	BELL
”	GELS
”	IGN
retention	BELL
”	CANTH
”	GELS
”	MAG-P
overexertion,	ARN
painful	ACON
”	APIS
”	CANTH
slow voiding	HEP
soreness with	APIS
sudden call	SULPH
suppression	ACON
”	FER-P
unfinished, feels like	HEP
urgency	CANTH

URINARY	
weakness after	ARS
wetting bed	CALC-P
"	FER-P
Urine	
albuminous	ARS
"	MERC
beer, like	BRY
bloody	ACON
"	CANTH
"	MERC
brown	BRY
"	PHOS
casts in	APIS
clear	GELS
colorless	SULPH
dark	BELL
"	MERC
"	PULS
fiery red	ACON
gravel	CALC-P
hot	ACON
"	BRY
jellylike	CANTH
mucus in	SULPH
muddy deposit	ACON
painful	ACON
pus in	SULPH
red	ALL-C
"	ARN
"	BELL
"	BRY
"	PHOS
retention, painful	ACON
"	APIS

URINARY	
,,	CANTH
scalding	APIS
,,	CANTH
scanty	ACON
,,	APIS
,,	ARS
,,	BELL
,,	BRY
,,	PULS
,,	PHOS
watery	GELS
,,	IGN
white sediment	RHUS

CHAPTER 13

Now Take a
Deep Breath and . . .

RESPIRATORY	
Asthma	IP
after eating	NUX
breathing in with	SPONG
chest oppressed	MAG-P
cold air, worsened by	SPONG
dampness, better with	HEP
discharge, nose	IP
drink, worsens	ARS
dry, cold air	HEP
elderly, in	CARB-V
foggy weather	HYPER
lying flat worsens	ARS
restlessness with	ARS
stomach full	NUX
walking improves	ARS
wheezing	ANT-T
”	ARS
Breathing	
difficult	ANT-T
“	APIS

RESPIRATORY	
hurried	APIS
labored	IP
moaning with	BELL
oppressed	ALL-C
”	BELL
”	GELS
”	NUX
”	PHOS
quick	BELL
”	GELS
”	PHOS
rapid	ANT-T
shallow	NUX
sighing	CALC-P
”	IGN
short	ANT-T
”	PULS
”	RUTA
shortness	ACON
suffocated	APIS
”	ARS
unequal	BELL
wheezing	HEP
Bronchitis	
acute	GELS
elderly, in	RHUS
”	VERAT-A
later	LED
Chest	
burning	ARS
constricted	IP
pain	ARS
pressure	ACON
stitches	BRY

RESPIRATORY

,,	CANTH
,,	PHOS
tightness	PHOS
,,	RUTA
touch, hurts	LED
Cough	
acute	FER-P
air, improved by open	PULS
anxiety with	PULS
asthma with	SPONG
back, while lying on	ARS
barking	BELL
,,	SPONG
,,	VERAT-A
bloody, expectorant	ACON
,,	ARN
,,	BELL
body trembles with	PHOS
choking	HEP
chronic	CALC-P
convulsive	CARB-V
,,	MAG-P
cold air, worse	ACON
,,	PHOS
cold foods, after eating	HEP
croupy	HEP
,,	FER-P
crying, causes	ARN
day & night	CHAM
day	HEP
dizziness with	ANT-T
drafts, worsen	PHOS
drinking, after	ARS
,,	BRY

RESPIRATORY	
,,	SPONG
dry	ACON
,,	BELL
,,	BRY
,,	CHAM
,,	FER-P
,,	HEP
,,	IP
,,	MERC
,,	NUX
,,	PHOS
,,	SULPH
earache, with	ALL-C
eating, worse	ANT-T
,,	BELL
,,	PHOS
evening in bed	CARB-V
exercise, worse	ARN
exhausting	IP
,,	NUX
first stage of	**FER-P**
frequent	ACON
,,	BRY
gagging	BRY
,,	IP
hacking	ALL-C
,,	BELL
hard	FER-P
headache with	NUX
hoarse	ANT-T
,,	APIS
,,	CHAM
hollow	BELL
incessant	IP

RESPIRATORY	
irritable	CHAM
laughter, worse	PHOS
left hip, pain	BELL
loose	PULS
,,	SULPH
lying down, improved by	BRY
,,	ALL-C
lying down, worse by	MAG-P
,,	SPONG
right side worse	MERC
midnight, before	SPONG
midnight, after	ACON
midnight to a.m.	RHUS
motion, worsened by	BRY
must sit up	BRY
,,	PULS
nausea with	IP
nervous	MAG-P
,,	PHOS
night, worsens	ACON
,,	BELL
night, improves	FER-P
nosebleed with	MERC
occasional	CARB-V
palpitation with	ANT-T
,,	HEP
,,	PULS
paroxysms	**IP**
,,	**NUX**
pleurisy with	BRY
racking	PHOS
rattling	ANT-T
,,	SULPH
,,	VERAT-A

RESPIRATORY	
reading, worse by	PHOS
short	ACON
"	FER-P
sleep, during	ARN
spasmodic	ARN
"	MAG-P
spells of	IGN
stomach, pain	BELL
feels like something strange is there	PHOS
suffocative	CALC-P
"	IP
talking worsens	PHOS
tickling	ACON
"	ARN
"	FER-P
urination with	PULS
"	VERAT-A
violent	ARN
"	MERC
"	IP
vomiting	IP
walking, worse by	HEP
warm room, worse in	BRY
"	PULS
"	VERAT-A
west wind, worse by	HEP
wheezing	ARS
whooping	CARB-V
"	IP
"	MAG-P
"	MERC
wind, cold	ACON
worse by	SPONG
yearly	IP

RESPIRATORY	
Croup	
first stage	ACON
"	FER-P
fear causes	IGN
fever with	BELL
hoarse cough with	SPONG
rattling	ANT-T
midnight, after	HEP
Emphysema in the elderly	ANT-T
"	LED
Hay Fever, fall & spring	**ALL-C**
open air, improves	**PULS**
sneezing	**ALL-C**
"	**ARS**
Influenza	
prevention	ARS
bones ache	RHUS
Pneumonia	ARN
"	FER-P
"	PHOS

CHAPTER 14

You've Got to Have Heart!

CIRCULATORY	
Angina pectoris	ARN
"	ARS
"	MAG-P
"	SPONG
Dilated heart	PHOS
Enlarged heart	ARN
from overexertion,	RHUS
especially right side	SPONG
Extremities, feel bruised	ARN
Fatty heart	ARN
"	ARS
Fear of death	SPONG
First stage of cardiac disease	FER-P
Liver, problems with	VERAT-A
Lie down, cannot	SPONG
Motion, necessary to keep in	GELS
Pain	ARS
elbow, left arm	ARN
constriction	MAG-P
left shoulder	ACON

CIRCULATORY	
midnight, after	SPONG
neck	ARS
occiput	ARS
stitching	ACON
Palpitation	**ARS**
”	**FER-P**
anxiety with	ACON
”	VERAT-A
least exertion	BELL
nervous	MAG-P
rapid	SPONG
sitting still	RHUS
spasmodic	MAG-P
violent	BELL
”	PHOS
”	SPONG
Pulse	
elderly, in	GELS
feeble	ARN
”	VERAT-A
full, all around	FER-P
full hard	ACON
irregular	ARN
”	RHUS
”	VERAT-A
rapid	FER-P
”	RHUS
”	ANT-T
”	PHOS
morning	ARS
weak	BELL
short, soft	FER-P
slow	GELS
soft	PHOS

CIRCULATORY	
weak	ANT-T
"	GELS
"	PHOS
Rapid heartbeat	ACON
Respiration heard	VERAT-A
Skin looks blue	ARS
Smoking worsens	ARS
Stimulant for	VERAT-A
Suffocation fear	SPONG
Throbbing, everywhere	BELL
Tingling fingers	ACON
Valvular, insufficency	SPONG
Warmth, feels in	PHOS

CHAPTER 15

Hats Off
to the Ladies!

FEMALE	
Breasts	
burning	CALC-P
enlarged	CALC-P
painful	MERC
stitching	PHOS
Discharge-Vaginal	
white, milky	CALC-P
mucusy	PULS
burning	ARS
"	SULPH
greenish	MERC
constant	CANTH
creamy	PULS
offensve odor	HEP
profuse	PHOS
yellow	CHAM
Frigidity	IGN
Infertility	PHOS
Labia, swollen	APIS
abscess	HEP

FEMALE	
Menstruation	
absence of	
agitation	BELL
asthma with	SPONG
due to chill	ACON
”	BRY
fright	BRY
grief	IG
backache with	CALC-P
”	PULS
before, worse	BELL
between, worse	BELL
black blood	NUX
”	PULS
bright red	BELL
”	IP
clotted	PULS
delayed start	SULPH
chill, from	ACON
fear, from	ACON
in young girls	**PULS**
nausea	VERAT-A
nose bleeds with	ACON
”	BRY
scanty, short	SULPH
diarrhea with	PULS
difficult, from coccyx injury	HYPER
early	ARS
”	BELL
”	BRY
”	IP
dark, stringy	MAG-P
lasts long	NUX
”	PHOS

FEMALE	
,,	RHUS
profuse	RHUS
excessive	ARS
,,	CALC-P
abdominal pains	MERC
after anger	CHAM
black	IGN
bright red blood	BELL
bowels, feel	NUX
clots with	CHAM
dark blood	CHAM
early	CARB-V
,,	RHUS
,,	VERAT-A
exhausting	VERAT-A
fainting with	APIS
,,	VERAT-A
irritation	CHAM
motion worsens	BRY
nausea	IP
pain stinging	APIS
restless with	PHOS
hands burn with	CARB-V
headache, before	SULPH
hunger, before	SPONG
intermittent, young girls	PULS
offensive odor	BELL
irregular	NUX
,,	PULS
,,	SULPH
painful	**CHAM**
,,	**MAG-P**
abdomen	GELS
angry	CHAM

FEMALE	
breasts with	BRY
burning	SULPH
clots	CHAM
cramps	MAG-P
day before	BELL
heat betters	MAG-P
in attacks	MAG-P
intense	PULS
labor-like	CHAM
lower back	GELS
lying down	BELL
red hot wires	ARS
sacrum	NUX
severe	APIS
scanty flow	GELS
sharp	GELS
shooting up	RHUS
thigh, down	ARS
unendurable	ACON
young girls	GELS
palpitation with	SPONG
scanty	IGN
chill, shock	ACON
dizziness	BRY
nervous	PHOS
thirst absent	PULS
soles burn with	CARB-V
sore throat with	GELS
stringy	MAG-P
suddenly stops	SULPH
suppressed	GELS
backache with	CALC-P
chill	ACON
grief	IGN

FEMALE	
headache with	BRY
wet feet	PULS
young girls	APIS
three weeks	FER-P
two weeks	CALC-P
voice lost with	GELS
wakes with suffocative spells	SPONG
variable	PHOS
"	PULS
Nipples cracked	SULPH
inflamed	CHAM
itching	HEP
Nymphomania	CALC-P
"	CANTH
"	PHOS
before menses	VERAT-A
Ovarian,	
neuralgia	MAG-P
tumors	APIS
Ovaritis,	APIS
burning pain	CANTH
especially right	BRY
stinging pain	MERC
Pregancy	
anemia while	CALC-P
"	FER-P
breast abscess,	
acute early	ACON
hard, tense	BRY
inflamed	BELL
breasts painful	PULS
"	BRY
heavy, red	BELL
excess milk	PULS

91

FEMALE	
insomnia,	
chills	ACON
craves food	PULS
2-5 a.m.	SULPH
lack of milk	
anger	CHAM
fear	ACON
labor, delayed	
dilation, no	BELL
false pains	GELS
pain unbearable	CHAM
weak contractions	NUX
”	PULS
labor, prolonged	
exhaustion	ARN
difficult	CHAM
painful	CHAM
”	GELS
mastitis	
acute, early	ACON
abcess, danger of	MERC
developed	HEP
burning pain	SULPH
hard	BRY
hot	BELL
injury	ARN
miscarriage, prevention of	
accident	ARN
disease	PHOS
hemorrhage	BELL
nerves	CHAM
third month	APIS
morning sickness	
”	IP

FEMALE	
"	MERC
"	NUX
movement of fetus	ARN
"	PULS
palpitations	NUX
placenta retained	CANTH
Pre-menstrual Tension or PMS	
Irritable	**NUX**
Painful	**PULS**
Weepy	**PULS**
Perspiration odor	SULPH
Pudenda, itching	HEP
"	SULPH
Sore nipples	ARN
Uterine,	
hemorrhages	CHAM
"	IP
"	PHOS
Uterus, polyps	PHOS
Uterus, prolapsus	NUX
Uterus, tender	APIS
Vagina	
burns	SULPH
dry	BELL
inflamed	MAG-P
sensitive	ACON
Vulva, swollen	CANTH
"	CARB-V
itching with	RHUS

CHAPTER 16

No Women Need Apply!

MALE	
Cold genitals	GELS
"	MERC
"	SULPH
Emissions	
backache with	NUX
involuntary	PHOS
"	SULPH
overindulgence	NUX
weakness	NUX
Erections	
emissions with	ACON
frequent	ACON
lack of power	PHOS
painful	ACON
"	CANTH
sperm eject, without	GELS
Figworts, without bad odor	HEP
Herpes, sensitive	HEP
Nightly emissions	
bloody	MERC

MALE	
dreams with	NUX
"	PHOS
Penis, end of	
crawling	ACON
itching	HEP
"	MERC
"	RHUS
painful	CANTH
stitches	SULPH
stinging	ACON
swelling	RHUS
Prostatic fluid,	
discharge with stool	CARB-V
flow of	BELL
Prostatitis,	
acute	**PULS**
Sexual desire	
diminished	BELL
easily aroused	NUX
excess	CANTH
bad effects	NUX
irresistible	PHOS
Testicles	
bruised	ACON
constrictive	NUX
drawn up	BELL
eczema	CANTH
hard	ACON
"	BELL
humid soreness	HEP
inflamed,	BELL
greatly	PULS
"	SPONG
itching,	HEP

MALE	
intense	RHUS
bedtime	SULPH
itching near	CARB-V
swollen	ACON
,,	NUX
,,	PULS
,,	RHUS
,,	SPONG
thigh, moist near	CARB-V
Urethra,	
yellow discharge	PULS
vesicles & ulcers	MERC

CHAPTER 17

The Anklebone is Connected to the . . .

BACK & EXTREMITIES	
Aching of limbs	CALC-P
Achilles, pain	IGN
"	RUTA
Ankles	
bone pain	RUTA
collapse	CHAM
sprain easily	**LED**
stiffness	SULPH
swollen	LED
Arms	
asleep, feel	NUX
loss of power	NUX
numbness	PHOS
sore, tired	ALL-C
swollen, feel	VERAT-A
Back	
asleep, feels	CALC-P
broken, feels	PHOS
bruised, feels	GELS
burning	PHOS

BACK & EXTREMITIES

center	ACON
coccyx, heavy	ANT-T
cold water improves	BRY
crawling	RHUS
crick in	FER-P
dislocated	ARN
draft worsens	CALC-P
fatigue, easy	GELS
injuries to	HYPER
mornings, worse in	CALC-P
numbness	ACON
overexertion	**ARN**
pain in	**ACON**
"	**ARS**
"	**CALC-P**
"	**FER-P**
"	**RUTA**
pressure improves	RUTA
rheumatic pain	APIS
shooting pain	PULS
sitting worsens	MERC
"	NUX
small of	
aches	GELS
broken, feels	CALC-P
morning pain	RUTA
pain	RHUS
"	BRY
"	NUX
shooting pain	PULS
violent pain	ANT-T
"	BELL
weakness in	ARS
sprained, feels	RHUS

BACK & EXTREMITIES	
stiff, feels	ACON
,,	RHUS
tingling	ACON
bed, worse in	CHAM
,,	LED
Bowlegs	CALC-P
Buttocks, asleep	CALC-P
Calves, cramps	**ARS**
,,	CALC-P
,,	MAG-P
,,	HYPER
,,	VERAT-A
pain in	IGN
Cold air worsens	RHUS
Cold, from knees down	CARB-V
Coccyx, injury to	HYPER
pain in	MERC
Elbow, numbness,	PULS
stitches in	PHOS
Feet	
cold	ACON
bone pains	RUTA
burning in	PHOS
dragged	NUX
hot	BRY
inflamed	PULS
misstep	ACON
night, worse at	CHAM
red	PULS
swollen	**APIS**
,,	ARS
,,	BRY
,,	MERC
,,	PULS

BACK & EXTREMITIES

tingling	RHUS
Fingers	
contract	RUTA
injured	HYPER
joints swollen	HEP
lose power	RHUS
numbness	APIS
tips, pain in	HYPER
stiff	MAG-P
Forearm	
cold	ARN
loses power	RHUS
veins swollen	PULS
Ganglion	RUTA
"	SULPH
Gout	ARN
"	CALC-P
"	FER-P
"	LED
with itching	SULPH
Hamstrings, short	RUTA
Hands	
burn at night	SULPH
can't hold anything	PHOS
drawing pain	SULPH
fall asleep	CALC-P
hot	ACON
"	SULPH
numbness	ACON
"	APIS
"	PHOS
painful	FER-P
palms hot	FER-P
shaking	MAG-P

BACK & EXTREMITIES

"	MERC
stiffness	RUTA
sweaty	SULPH
swollen	FER-P
tingling	ACON
veins swell	PULS
Heel, boring pain	PULS
ulcer on	ALL-C
"	ARS
Hip	
insupportble	CHAM
joint, lame	ACON
painful	BELL
"	GELS
"	PULS
weakness in	RUTA
Hives	APIS
Hysteric spasms	GELS
Joints	
bruised, feel	HYPER
crack	ACON
"	LED
give way	PHOS
inflamed	ACON
lame	ALL-C
movement worsens	BRY
painful	CALC-P
"	RHUS
"	VERAT-A
red	ACON
"	BRY
swollen	ACON
"	BRY
"	RHUS

BACK & EXTREMITIES

weak	ACON
Knee	
cracking in	NUX
painful	BRY
stiff	BRY
"	SULPH
swollen	APIS
"	CALC-P
"	PULS
tender	RHUS
unsteady	ACON
Left arm & leg, constant motion	BRY
Legs	
give way	RUTA
heavy, feel	PULS
loss of power	NUX
numbness	NUX
swollen	MERC
weary, feel	PULS
Limbs	
asleep	CARB-V
burning	CARB-V
cold	CALC-P
painful	PULS
paralyzed	ARS
"	CARB-V
"	RHUS
stiff	RHUS
weakness	MERC
Muscles	
jerking	HYPER
loss of control	GELS
"	NUX
twitching	ANT-T

BACK & EXTREMITIES	
,,	HYPER
weakness in	MAG-P
Nails	
infected	ALL-C
,,	FER-P
large toe pain	HEP
root pain	CALC-P
Neck, nape	
painful	BELL
,,	BRY
,,	HYPER
shooting pain	PULS
stiff	BELL
,,	CHAM
,,	FER-P
,,	RHUS
,,	SULPH
swollen glands	BELL
Neuralgia	HYPER
Numbness	CALC-P
overwork, from	RHUS
Paralysis	MAG-P
,,	MERC
Restlessness, great	RUTA
Rheumatism	
begins lower limbs	LED
pain all over	RHUS
Right side, can only lie on	PHOS
Sciatica	
,,	ARS
,,	MAG-P
cold worsens	RHUS
dampness worsens	RHUS
electric flashes	VERAT-A

BACK & EXTREMITIES

evening, worse in the	RUTA
lying down worsens	RUTA
Shin bones, pain	CALC-P
"	CARB-V
Shoulders	
heat between	PHOS
left, pain in	SULPH
pain	FER-P
"	HYPER
pain between	SULPH
pain/swallowing	RHUS
Soles of feet	
burn at night	**CANTH**
"	CHAM
"	SULPH
cramps in	CARB-V
painful	CANTH
"	IGN
throbbing in	LED
spasms	ARS
"	IP
Spine, trauma	HYPER
weak	PHOS
Stoop-shouldered	SULPH
Stretched stiff	IP
Sweat underarm, garlic odor	SULPH
Synovitis	APIS
Thigh	
lame, feels	ACON
painful	BELL
"	CANTH
"	CHAM
stretch, worse	RUTA
tearing down	RHUS

BACK & EXTREMITIES

water trickle	ACON
weakness in	RUTA
Tibia, inflamed	PHOS
Toes	
ball of big toe	LED
tips, pain in	HYPER
red, swollen	CARB-V
Trembling	ARS
Walking,	
not erect	ARN
slowness	CALC-P
Weather change worsens	BRY
Wet feet worsens	ALL-C
Wrist, painful	RUTA
Writer's Cramp	**GELS**
"	**MAG-P**

CHAPTER 18

What You See is What You Are!

SKIN	
Abscesses	HEP
Acne	
in youths	HEP
,,	PULS
on forehead	LED
red, blotchy	NUX
Bed sores	ARN
Bleeds easily	PHOS
Blisters, blue	CARB-V
Blue,	CARB-V
,,	VERAT-A
around eyes	IP
Blue-red mark	ANT-T
Boils,	BELL
crops of	ARN
Brownish-red	ACON
Bruises	
black & blue	ARN
,,	LED
nerve, injury to	HYPER

SKIN	
Burning	ACON
,,	ARN
,,	ARS
Burning hot, body	NUX
Burning in spots	PULS
Burns, scalds	CANTH
Carbuncle	APIS
,,	CARB-V
Cervical, glands swollen	SPONG
Chafing, infants	ARN
,,	CHAM
,,	MERC
,,	SULPH
Chapped	HEP
Chicken pox	
after fever	MERC
during fever	ACON
Cold	CARB-V
clammy	VERAT-A
death-like	VERAT-A
worse	ARS
Coldsores	**HEP**
Cracks, hands/feet	HEP
Dermatitis	CANTH
Diaper rash,	
chilly baby	HEP
hot baby	SULPH
restless baby	ACON
,,	CHAM
Discoloration, after injury	LED
Draught, sensitive to	IGN
Dropsical	BRY
Dry	ACON
,,	BELL

SKIN	
,,	PULS
Eczema, facial	LED
genitals	CANTH
Eruption	CARB-V
,,	PULS
,,	SULPH
cold water improves	PULS
eating fats, from	PULS
pork	PULS
Flabby	ARS
Freckles	CALC-C
Fungus infections	**PHOS**
Gangrene, tend to	CANTH
senile	CARB-V
Glands swell/colds	MERC
Hair	
falls out,	CARB-V
after injury	HYPER
very greasy	BRY
Hard patches	ARS
,,	RHUS
Herpes	HEP
Hives,	**ARS**
chronic	HEP
delay of menses	PULS
gastric,	NUX
rich foods	PULS
Hot	ACON
,,	BELL
,,	BRY
,,	PULS
Icy cold	VERAT-A
Induration, after inflammation	BELL
Inflammation	RHUS

SKIN	
Itching	ACON
,,	ARN
,,	ARS
,,	CALC-P
,,	IGN
,,	SPONG
evening worsens	CARB-V
feet & ankles	LED
intense	RHUS
warmth of bed	MERC
Jaundice	PHOS
Lax	IP
Leaden color	MERC
Loose	ARS
Marbled, looks	CARB-V
Measles	**FER-P**
,,	PULS
,,	SPONG
bring out rash	GELS
chest affected	PHOS
diarrhea after	PULS
fever	ACON
,,	SULPH
rash,	ANT-T
burning after	ARS
,,	SULPH
itching	ARS
,,	SULPH
respiratory, with	BRY
skin tender, after	RHUS
vomiting after	ARS
,,	CHAM
Moist constantly	MERC
Nettle-rash	IGN

SKIN	
Odor, rotten eggs	SULPH
Pale	BRY
Patches, raised	RHUS
Perspiration	
cold, clammy	VERAT-A
day & night	HEP
freely	MERC
hot	CARB-V
Poison Ivy	**LED**
”	**RHUS**
Pricking, feels	HEP
Prickling,	PULS
heat	ACON
”	BRY
”	CHAM
”	SULPH
Purple	ACON
Pustular, blue-red	ANT-T
Red,	ACON
spots	PULS
Redness and pale, alternating	BELL
Rough	ARS
Seborrhea	BRY
Sensitive	BELL
Scabs	RHUS
Scalds, burns	CANTH
Scaly	ARS
”	RHUS
Scalp sweats	MERC
Scarlet fever	GELS
scratching, worse	LED
Scurfy patches	ARS
Shingles	**HYPER**
Smallpox	ANT-T

SKIN	
"	HEP
Stuck, feels like being	HEP
Stings	
bee	**APIS**
infected	**CANTH**
insects	**LED**
wasps	**ARN**
Stinging pain	APIS
Strep infection	BELL
Sunburn	CANTH
Swollen	ACON
"	ARS
"	BRY
esp. after bites	APIS
Ulcers	ARN
bleeding	PHOS
cheese smell	HEP
discharge	ARS
indolent	CARB-V
irregular shape	MERC
sensitive to touch	HEP
varicose	CARB-V
Unhealthy varicose veins	PULS
Warm bed worsens	LED
"	MERC
Warts	**ANT-T**
Wounds, lacerated	HYPER
Wrapped up improves	HEP
Yellow,	BRY
in newborn	MERC

CHAPTER 19

For the Rip Van Winkle in Us All!

SLEEP	
Afternoon, sleepy	PULS
Anxiety in chest	ACON
Anxious	ARS
Awakens	
frequently	SULPH
in a fright	SPONG
with hot head	ARN
Singing, to find self	SULPH
slight noise	SULPH
Cannot fall into	GELS
Cannot sleep after	
3 a.m. to morning	NUX
2 a.m. to 5 a.m.	SULPH
Catnaps	SULPH
Comotose	ARN
Crying out in	BELL
"	CALC-P
Delirium	BRY
"	GELS
Disturbed	ARS

SLEEP	
Dreams	ALL-C
anxious	ACON
,,	ARN
,,	FER-P
bustle, hurry	NUX
care & toil	APIS
death	ARN
fear	ARS
fire	PHOS
frightening	CHAM
great exertion	RHUS
long	ACON
,,	IGN
sexual	PHOS
upsetting	IGN
vivid	SULPH
Drowsiness, great	**ANT-T**
,,	**APIS**
,,	**ARS**
with sleeplessness	BELL
after meals	**NUX**
,,	**PHOS**
with moaning	**CHAM**
early evening	NUX
Electric shocks,	
on falling asleep	ANT-T
,,	IP
Eyes half open	CHAM
,,	IP
Exhausted after	SPONG
Grinding teeth	BELL
Hands,	
over head, with	ARS
,,	PULS

SLEEP	
under head	BELL
Heavy, stuporlike	RHUS
Horrors in night	ARN
Insomnia	
elderly, in	ACON
"	PHOS
from exhaustion	GELS
from grief	IGN
smoking	GELS
thinking	GELS
Involuntary stool	ARN
Irresistible need	ANT-T
Jerks, when	
falling asleep	BELL
"	IGN
closing eyes	BRY
during sleep	SULPH
Nightmares	**ACON**
Night sweats	FER-P
Noise awakens	SULPH
Pillows, extra required	ARS
Pulse keeps awake	BELL
Restless,	ARS
"	FER-P
when overtired	ARN
Screams out	APIS
Short naps,	
improves	NUX
frequent wakings	PHOS
Sleeping sickness	ARS
Sleeplessness	ACON
"	FER-P
before midnight	RHUS
nervous tension	GELS

SLEEP	
when overtired	ARN
with drowsiness	BELL
Suffocated, feels	SPONG
Talks in	SULPH
Tired, awakens	PHOS
"	PULS
Tosses about	ACON
Twitches during	SULPH
Very light	IGN
Wakes at 2 a.m.	ALL-C
weeping, wailing	CHAM
Wide awake,	
in evening	PULS
suddenly	SULPH
Work, thinks about	BRY
Yawning,	GELS
drowsiness	ALL-C
headaches	ALL-C

CHAPTER 20

There Will Be
a Hot Time . . .

FEVER	
Afternoon chill	APIS
Anxiety with heat	SPONG
Blueness: nails	NUX
Burning	
intolerable	PULS
various places	CARB-V
Chilliness	ANT-T
after dinner	MAG-P
at 1 p.m.	FER-P
at 4 p.m.	PULS
forearm	CARB-V
open air	HEP
up/down back	MAG-P
with thirst	IGN
without thirst	PULS
Cold knees, evenings	PHOS
Cold & hot altnernating	ACON
Coldness	ANT-T
extreme	VERAT-A
no body heat	LED

FEVER	
with thirst	CARB-V
Cold water over,	
feels like	CANTH
,,	LED
,,	RHUS
Covered, must be	NUX
Delirium with	ARS
Stupor	PHOS
Evening chillness	ACON
,,	PHOS
Exhaustion from	ARS
,,	CARB-V
Face, red & hot	SPONG
Feet, icy cold	BELL
First stage of fever	**ACON**
,,	**FER-P**
Gastric, bilious	MERC
Hands/feet cold	CANTH
Head hot & red, body cold	ARN
Heat	
about 3 a.m.	ARS
dry, night	HEP
flashes of	SULPH
worsened by	APIS
High temperature	ARS
,,	BELL
hot & cold alternating	ACON
intermittent	ARS
,,	IP
,,	RHUS
Itching with	IGN
Lethargy, alternating with	ANT-T
Midnight, worse after	ARS
Motion, worsened by	APIS

FEVER	
Muscle soreness	GELS
,,	NUX
Nausea with	IP
Nettle-rash with	IGN
Nightly sweats	ARN
,,	MERC
Pulse	
quick, small	PHOS
rapid	BRY
slow	GELS
Restlessness	ACON
,,	RHUS
Shivering all over	ARN
,,	MAG-P
Sleepy after fever	APIS
Soles, feet burn	CANTH
Stretch, wants to	RHUS
Sweat	
cold	ARS
cold & clammy	ANT-T
cold & icy	ACON
disgusting	SULPH
drenches	ACON
exhausting	CARB-V
,,	GELS
face red & hot	SPONG
night, viscid	PHOS
one side body	NUX
,,	PULS
pains with	PULS
profuse	HEP
,,	MERC
,,	PHOS
single parts	SULPH

FEVER	
slight	APIS
sour, in a.m.	NUX
sour, after exercise	BRY
sour, nightly	ARN
"	HEP
Thirst	VERAT-A
great	ACON
"	APIS
"	SULPH
absent	BELL
"	GELS
Trembling	ACON
"	RHUS
Veins distended	PULS
Wants to be held	GELS

CHAPTER 21

Ready . . . Fire . . . Aim!

MODALITIES

If you feel dis-eased *after* doing any of the following, i.e., eating, drinking, being out in the open air, etc., the remedies indicated will help correct this condition.

"First Choice" remedies are indicated by "**", "Second Choice" by a single * and "Third Choice" by no asterisk.

This is a good way to successfully treat many food allergies.

FEELING DIS-EASED BY:	
Acids (sour) foods	ACON**
"	ANT-T
"	APIS
"	ARS*
"	BELL*
"	CARB-V**
"	HEP**
"	IP
"	NUX
"	PHOS

FEELING DIS-EASED BY:	
,,	PULS*
,,	RHUS*
,,	SULPH*
Afternoon	ARS
,,	BELL*
,,	RHUS*
Afternoon, late	APIS
,,	PULS
Air, cold, dry	ARS
,,	BELL
,,	BRY
,,	CHAM
,,	IGN
,,	NUX
"	SPONG
Air, open	ACON
,,	BRY
,,	CHAM*
,,	IGN
,,	NUX*
Alcohol, drinking	ACON
,,	ARS*
,,	BELL
,,	CARB-V
,,	GELS
,,	HEP
,,	IGN
,,	IP
,,	LED
,,	MERC
,,	NUX*
,,	PHOS
,,	PULS
,,	RHUS

FEELING DIS-EASED BY:	
,,	RUTA
,,	SULPH*
Ale, drinking	SPONG
,,	SULPH
Anger, after	**BRY**
,,	CHAM
,,	IGN
,,	NUX
Antibiotics, after using	**NUX**
Apples, eating	ANT-T
,,	ARS
,,	PHOS
,,	PULS
,,	SULPH
Aromatic drinks	PULS
Ascending stairs	ARS*
,,	SPONG
Autumn	MERC
Bathing	MAG-P
,,	NUX
,,	RHUS*
,,	SULPH*
Beans, eating	ARS
,,	BRY*
,,	PHOS
,,	PULS
,,	SULPH
Bed, turning in	NUX
,,	PULS
Beer, drinking	ACON
,,	ARS
,,	BELL
,,	BRY*
,,	IGN

FEELING DIS-EASED BY:	
"	LED*
"	NUX**
"	PULS
"	RHUS*
Bending forward	BELL*
"	NUX
Bitter drinks	ACON
Brandy (cognac)	ARS*
"	BELL
"	HEP
"	IGN
"	LED*
"	NUX**
"	PULS
"	RHUS*
"	RUTA
"	SULPH**
Bread, eating	BRY**
"	MERC
"	NUX
"	PHOS
"	PULS**
"	RHUS*
"	RUTA
"	SULPH
Breakfast, after	CHAM
"	NUX*
"	PHOS
Breathing in	ACON*
"	BRY*
"	PHOS
Bright objects	BELL
"	CANTH
Buckwheat, eating	IP

FEELING DIS-EASED BY:	
,,	PHOS*
,,	PULS**
,,	VERAT-A
Butter, eating	ACON
,,	ANT-T
,,	ARS*
,,	BELL
,,	CARB-V**
,,	HEP
,,	IP
,,	NUX
,,	PHOS*
,,	PULS**
,,	SPONG
,,	SULPH
Buttermilk	PULS
Cabbage, eating	ARS
,,	BRY**
,,	CARB-V
,,	PHOS
,,	PULS*
,,	SULPH
Carbohydrates	BRY*
,,	CARB-V
,,	NUX
,,	PULS**
,,	SULPH
Cheese, eating	ARS
,,	NUX
,,	PHOS
Chicken, eating	BRY
Chocolate, eating	BRY
,,	PULS*
Cider, drinking	PHOS

FEELING DIS-EASED BY:	
Coffee, drinking	ARS
,,	BELL
,,	BRY
,,	CALC-P*
,,	CANTH**
,,	CARB-V
,,	CHAM**
,,	HEP
,,	IGN**
,,	IP
,,	MERC
,,	NUX**
,,	PULS*
,,	RHUS
,,	SULPH
Cold, being	ACON*
,,	ARS
,,	BELL
,,	BRY*
,,	CHAM
,,	HEP
,,	IGN
,,	MAG-P*
,,	NUX*
,,	RHUS*
,,	RUTA
Cold food, eating	ACON
,,	ARS**
,,	BELL*
,,	BRY*
,,	CALC-P*
,,	CANTH
,,	CARB-V*
,,	CHAM

FEELING DIS-EASED BY:	
"	HEP*
"	IP
"	MAG-P
"	MERC*
"	NUX**
"	PULS*
"	RHUS**
"	SULPH*
Cold water, drink	APIS
"	BELL*
"	CALC-P
"	CANTH**
"	CARB-V*
"	CHAM
"	FER-P
"	HEP
"	IGN*
"	MAG-P*
"	MERC
"	NUX*
"	RHUS**
"	SPONG
"	SULPH*
Cooked food	ARS
Consolation	IGN
Corn, eating	PULS
"	SULPH
Cough, after	ARS
"	BRY
"	PHOS*
Crying, after	CHAM
"	PULS
Cucumbers, eating	ALL-C*
"	ARS

FEELING DIS-EASED BY:	
,,	PULS
Damp houses, in	ANT-T
,,	ARS
Dampness, in air	CARB-V
,,	RHUS*
,,	RUTA
,,	SULPH
Damp cold air, in	ANT-T
,,	ARN
,,	CALC-P*
,,	GELS
,,	NUX
,,	RHUS*
Dampness warm	CARB-V
,,	GELS*
,,	PHOS
Dark	ARS*
,,	PHOS
Dinner, after	ARS
,,	NUX*
Drinking, during	BELL
Dry food, eating	IGN
,,	IP
,,	NUX
,,	PULS*
,,	SULPH
Eggs, eating	PULS*
,,	SULPH
Eating, after	ARS*
,,	BRY*
,,	IGN
,,	IP*
,,	PHOS
,,	PULS*

FEELING DIS-EASED BY:	
,,	SULPH
Emotions, display	ACON
,,	GELS*
Emotions, display	IGN*
,,	NUX
,,	PHOS*
Erratic symptoms	APIS
,,	IGN*
,,	PULS*
Evening, during	ACON*
,,	ANT-T
,,	ARN
,,	BELL
,,	BRY
,,	CARB-V
,,	CHAM
,,	FER-P
,,	MERC*
,,	PHOS*
,,	PULS*
,,	RUTA
Eyes, after closing	BRY
Eyes, motion of	BRY*
,,	NUX
Fats, eating	ACON
,,	ANT-T
,,	ARS*
,,	CARB-V**
,,	HEP
,,	IP*
,,	NUX
,,	PHOS
,,	PULS**
,,	RUTA

FEELING DIS-EASED BY:	
,,	SPONG*
,,	SULPH*
Fish, eating	ARS
,,	CARB-V
,,	PULS*
Feet hang down	PULS
Fog, during	GELS
,,	HYPER
Fright, after	ACON*
,,	GELS
,,	IGN*
Frozen food, eating	ARS*
,,	BRY
,,	CARB-V*
,,	IP*
,,	PULS**
Fruit, eating	ACON
,,	ANT-T
,,	ARS**
,,	BRY**
,,	CARB-V
,,	IGN
,,	IP*
,,	MERC
,,	PHOS
,,	PULS**
,,	RUTA
,,	SULPH
Gassy foods	ARS
,,	BRY*
,,	CARB-V
,,	PULS
Grief, after	GELS
,,	IGN*

FEELING DIS-EASED BY:	
Haircut	ACON
"	BELL*
Head, uncovering	BELL
Honey, eating	PHOS
Hot drinks	APIS
"	BELL*
"	BRY**
"	CARB-V*
"	CHAM*
"	IGN
"	PHOS**
"	PULS**
Hot foods	ACON
"	ANT-T*
"	APIS
"	BELL*
"	BRY*
"	CARB-V
"	CHAM
"	MERC*
"	NUX
"	PHOS**
"	PULS*
"	RHUS
"	SULPH
Ice, food & drink	ARS**
"	BELL
"	BRY*
"	CALC-P
"	CARB-V**
"	HEP
"	IP
"	NUX*
"	PULS*

FEELING DIS-EASED BY:	
,,	RHUS
Ice cream, eating	ARS
,,	PULS
Jarred, being	ARN
,,	BELL*
,,	BRY*
,,	IGN
,,	NUX
Laughing	PHOS
Light	ACON
,,	BELL*
,,	IGN
,,	NUX*
,,	PHOS*
Liquors	ARS
,,	BELL
,,	CARB-V
,,	LED
,,	NUX*
,,	RHUS
,,	SULPH
,,	VERAT-A
Localized spots	IGN
Looking downwards	ACON
,,	SULPH
Looking upwards	PULS*
,,	SULPH
Lying down	ANT-T
,,	ARN
,,	BELL*
,,	IP
,,	PHOS*
,,	PULS*
,,	RHUS

Homeopathy Made Simple

FEELING DIS-EASED BY:	
,,	RUTA
Lying on back	NUX
,,	PULS
,,	RHUS
Lying, left side	PHOS*
,,	PULS
Lying, painful side	ACON
,,	ARS
,,	HEP*
,,	PHOS*
,,	RUTA
Lying, on painless side	BRY*
,,	CHAM
,,	PULS*
Lying on right side	MERC
,,	RHUS
Lying with head low	ARS
Masturbation	NUX
Meat, eating	ARS*
,,	BRY*
,,	CARB-V
,,	FER-P
,,	MERC
,,	NUX
,,	PULS*
,,	RUTA
,,	SULPH
,,	VERAT-A
Medication, excess	**NUX**
Menses, after	NUX
Menses, before	GELS*
Menses, before	PULS
Menses, during	BELL*
,,	CHAM

FEELING DIS-EASED BY:	
,,	NUX*
,,	PULS*
,,	SULPH
Mental exertion	GELS*
,,	IGN
,,	NUX
,,	PHOS*
Midnight, after	APIS
,,	ARS*
,,	BELL
,,	NUX*
,,	PHOS
,,	RHUS
Midnight, at	ARS
Midnight, before	CHAM,
,,	LED
,,	MERC*
,,	PHOS
,,	PULS*
,,	RHUS*
,,	SPONG*
Milk, drinking	ANT-T
,,	ARS*
,,	BRY
,,	CARB-V*
,,	CHAM*
,,	NUX*
,,	PHOS*
,,	RHUS
,,	SPONG
,,	SULPH**
Morning	BRY*
,,	IGN
,,	NUX*

FEELING DIS-EASED BY:	
,,	PHOS*
,,	PULS*
,,	RHUS
,,	SULPH*
Morning, early (2-5 a.m.)	BELL
,,	NUX*
Morning, (10-11 a.m.)	GELS
,,	SULPH
Motion	BELL*
,,	FER-P
,,	GELS
,,	IP
,,	LED*
,,	MAG-P
,,	NUX*
,,	PHOS
,,	RUTA
,,	SULPH
Motion downward	GELS
Motion, start of	PULS
,,	RHUS*
Mountain climbing	ARS
Music	ACON*
,,	NUX
Narcotics, use	BELL
,,	CHAM*
,,	NUX*
Night	ACON*
,,	ANT-T
,,	ARS*
"	BELL
,,	BRY
,,	CHAM*
,,	FER-P

FEELING DIS-EASED BY:	
,,	HEP*
,,	MAG-P
,,	MERC*
,,	PHOS*
,,	PULS*
,,	RHUS*
,,	SULPH
Noise	ACON
"	BELL*
,,	CHAM
,,	IGN*
,,	NUX*
,,	PHOS
Oil, foods cooked	BRY
,,	PULS*
One half of body	CHAM*
,,	IGN
,,	PULS*
Onions, eating	ACON
,,	NUX
,,	PULS*
Overeating	NUX*
,,	PULS
Overheating	ACON*
,,	ANT-T
,,	BELL*
,,	BRY*
,,	CARB-V
,,	NUX*
Oysters, eating	BRY
,,	CARB-V
,,	PULS*
Pancakes, eating	BRY*
,,	IP

FEELING DIS-EASED BY:	
,,	PULS**
,,	VERAT-A
Pastry, eating	ARS
,,	BRY*
,,	CARB-V
,,	IP
,,	PHOS*
,,	PULS**
,,	SULPH
,,	VERAT-A*
Pears	BRY
,,	VERAT-A*
Pepper	ARS
,,	NUX*
periodically	ARS*
,,	IGN
,,	IP
every 2-4 weeks	SULPH
every 3 weeks	ARS
every year	ARS
,,	SULPH
Pickles, eating	APIS
,,	ARS
,,	VERAT-A
Plums, eating	MERC*
,,	PULS
Pork, eating	ACON
,,	ANT-T
,,	ARS
,,	BELL
,,	CARB-V**
,,	IP*
,,	PULS**
Potatoes, eating	BRY*

FEELING DIS-EASED BY:	
,,	MERC
,,	PULS*
,,	SULPH*
,,	VERAT-A*
Pressure (touch)	ACON
,,	APIS*
,,	HEP
,,	MERC
,,	NUX*
Raw foods, eating	ARS
,,	BRY
,,	PULS*
,,	RUTA**
,,	VERAT-A*
Rest	ACON
,,	ARS*
,,	MERC*
,,	PULS*
"	RHUS*
Rice, eating	BRY
,,	PULS
,,	SULPH
Right side	BELL*
,,	BRY*
,,	FER-P
,,	MAG-P*
,,	MERC*
,,	RHUS
Rising, upon	ACON*
,,	BELL
,,	BRY*
,,	CARB-V
,,	NUX*
,,	PHOS

FEELING DIS-EASED BY:	
,,	PULS
,,	RHUS*
,,	SULPH
Room, heated	ACON
,,	APIS*
,,	ALL-C*
,,	HYPER
,,	MERC*
,,	PULS*
Salad, eating	ARS
,,	BRY
,,	CARB-V
,,	IP
,,	NUX
,,	PULS*
,,	SULPH
Salt, eating	ARS
,,	BELL
,,	CARB-V*
,,	NUX
,,	PHOS**
,,	PULS
Sauerkraut	ARS
,,	BRY**
,,	CARB-V
,,	PHOS*
,,	PULS*
,,	VERAT-A
Sausage, eating	ARS**
,,	BELL
,,	BRY
,,	PULS
Scratching, by	ARS
,,	MERC*

FEELING DIS-EASED BY:	
,,	PULS*
,,	RHUS
,,	SULPH
Sea, bathing in	ARS
Seashore, at	ARS
Sedentary habits	ACON
,,	BRY
,,	NUX*
Sex, after	NUX
,,	PHOS
Shellfish, eating	BELL
,,	CARB-V
,,	RHUS
Sight of food	ANT-T
,,	SULPH*
Sitting	BRY*
,,	NUX
,,	PULS
,,	RHUS*
,,	SULPH
Sitting on cold steps	NUX
Sleep, after	APIS*
,,	RHUS
,,	SPONG*
,,	SULPH
Smell of food	ARS*
,,	BELL
,,	IP*
,,	NUX
,,	PHOS
,,	SULPH
Smoking	GELS*
,,	IGN*
,,	NUX*

FEELING DIS-EASED BY:	
,,	PULS
Sneezing	ARS*
,,	PHOS
,,	SULPH*
Snow melting	CALC-P
Spices, eating	NUX*
,,	PHOS
Spring, in the	GELS
,,	RHUS
Standing	SULPH
Stimulants	IGN
,,	LED
,,	NUX*
Storm, before	RHUS
Stooping, by	BRY
,,	SULPH*
Straining from overlifting	RHUS*
,,	RUTA
Stretching	RHUS
Sugar, eating	BELL
,,	SULPH*
Sun, exposure	BELL*
,,	BRY
,,	GELS*
,,	PULS
Swallowing, by	APIS
,,	BELL*
,,	BRY
,,	HEP*
,,	MERC*
,,	SULPH
Sweating	ANT-T
,,	HEP*
Sweets, eating	ACON

FEELING DIS-EASED BY:	
,,	ARS
,,	BELL
,,	CHAM*
,,	HEP
,,	IGN**
,,	IP*
,,	MERC*
,,	NUX
,,	PHOS
,,	PULS*
,,	SPONG
,,	SULPH*
Talking	RHUS
"	SULPH
Tea, drinking	ARS
,,	CHAM
,,	HEP
,,	NUX*
,,	PULS
,,	RHUS*
Temperature, extremes of	IP
Teething, after	BELL*
,,	CALC-P
,,	CHAM*
Thinking of symptoms	CALC-P*
,,	GELS*
"	NUX
Thought of food	CARB-V
,,	PULS*
Thunderstorm,	
before, during	GELS
,,	PHOS*
Tobacco smoke	ACON
,,	IGN

FEELING DIS-EASED BY:	
Tomatoes	PHOS
Touched, being	ACON*
"	APIS*
"	BELL*
"	BRY*
"	CHAM*
"	HEP*
"	IGN
"	NUX*
"	PHOS
"	PULS
"	RHUS
"	SULPH
Turnips, eating	BRY*
"	PULS*
"	SULPH
Uncovering self	ARS
"	BELL
"	HEP*
"	MAG-P*
"	NUX*
"	RHUS*
Veal, eating	ARS
"	IP*
"	NUX
"	VERAT-A
Vegetables	ARS
"	BRY*
"	VERAT-A
Vinegar	ACON*
"	ARS*
"	BELL*
"	CARB-V*
"	HEP

FEELING DIS-EASED BY:	
,,	NUX
,,	PULS*
,,	SULPH*
Voice, using	CARB-V
,,	NUX
,,	PHOS*
Vomiting	ANT-T
,,	ARS*
,,	IP*
,,	NUX*
,,	PULS
Waking	NUX
Warm drinks	APIS
,,	BRY
,,	IGN
,,	PHOS*
,,	PULS*
,,	RHUS**
,,	SULPH*
Warm food, eating	ACON
,,	ANT-T
,,	ARS
,,	BELL*
,,	BRY**
,,	CANTH
,,	CARB-V*
,,	CHAM*
,,	NUX
,,	PHOS**
,,	PULS**
,,	RHUS*
,,	SULPH
Warmth, heat	ACON
,,	ANT-T

FEELING DIS-EASED BY:	
"	APIS*
"	BELL
"	BRY*
"	CHAM*
"	GELS
"	LED*
"	MERC*
"	PULS*
"	SULPH
Warmth, bed	APIS
"	CHAM*
"	LED*
"	MERC*
"	PULS*
"	SULPH*
Washing, water	BELL
"	CANTH
"	CHAM
"	MERC*
"	RHUS
"	SULPH
Water, drinking	
cold	ARS*
"	CANTH*
"	RHUS*
"	SPONG
"	SULPH
Water, drinking	
warm	BRY
"	PHOS
"	PULS*
Weather changes	BRY
"	CALC-P*
"	MERC*

FEELING DIS-EASED BY:	
,,	PHOS*
,,	RHUS*
,,	SULPH
Weather changes,	
in Spring	ANT-T
,,	GELS
Weather, dry cold	IP
,,	NUX*
,,	RHUS
Weather, hot	ACON*
,,	BELL*
,,	BRY*
,,	GELS*
,,	PHOS
,,	PULS
Weather stormy	RHUS
Weather,	ACON*
windy, dry	CHAM
,,	HEP*
,,	NUX*
,,	PHOS
,,	PULS
Weather,	
windy, moist	ALL-C
,,	IP
Wet applications	MERC*
,,	RHUS
,,	SULPH*
Wet exposure	APIS
,,	ARS
,,	ALL-C
,,	MERC*
,,	RHUS
,,	RUTA

FEELING DIS-EASED BY:	
Wet feet	ALL-C
,,	PULS
,,	RHUS*
Wine, drinking	ACON
,,	ARN*
,,	ARS**
,,	BELL
,,	BRY
,,	CARB-V*
,,	IGN
,,	LED*
,,	MERC*
,,	NUX**
,,	PHOS
,,	PULS
,,	RHUS
,,	RUTA
,,	SULPH*
,,	VERAT-A
Yawning	IGN*
,,	NUX*
,,	RHUS

If you feel better, or improved, *after* doing any of the following, the remedies indicated below will help correct the illness you are treating.

FEELING BETTER BY:	
Air, cool, open	ACON*
"	ANT-T
"	APIS*
"	BRY
"	ALL-C*
"	GELS
"	PHOS
"	PULS*
"	RHUS
Air, cool: must have windows open	PULS
"	SULPH
Air warm	LED
"	MERC
"	RHUS
Bathing	ACON
"	APIS
"	PULS*
Bathing, cold water	APIS
Belching	ANT-T
"	BRY
"	CARB-V
"	IGN
"	NUX
Bending double	MAG-P
Bending forward	GELS
Breathing in	IGN
Carried, being	ANT-T
"	CHAM*
Chewing	BRY

FEELING BETTER BY:	
Cold (weather)	ALL-C
,,	BRY*
,,	LED*
,,	PHOS*
Cold, applications	APIS*
,,	BELL
,,	FER-P
,,	PHOS
,,	PULS*
Consolation	PULS
Coughing	APIS
Dark	PHOS
Descending	SPONG
Drawing limbs up	SULPH
Drinks, warm	ARS
,,	NUX
,,	SPONG*
Eating	HEP*
,,	IGN*
,,	PHOS
,,	SPONG*
Evenings	NUX
Exercise	RHUS
Expectoration	ANT-T
,,	HEP
Flatulence	ARN
,,	CALC-P
,,	HEP
Fanned, being	CARB-V
Fasting	CHAM
Feet in ice water	LED
Food, cold	BRY
,,	PHOS
Head bent backward	HYPER

FEELING BETTER BY:	
Head, wrapped up	HEP
Head, elevated	ARS
,,	GELS
Heat	ARS*
Hypnotized, being	PHOS
Lying down	ACON
,,	ARN
,,	BELL*
,,	BRY*
,,	NUX
,,	PULS*
Lying on back	ACON
,,	ARS
Lying, left side	IGN
Lying, painful side	ARN
,,	BRY*
,,	PULS*
Lying, right side	ANT-T
,,	PHOS*
,,	SULPH
Lying, right side, head elevated	ARS
,,	SPONG
Lying, on stomach	ANT-T
Lying, head high	PULS
Lying, head low	ARN
,,	SPONG
Menses, between	BELL
Menses, during	BELL
Midnight to noon	PULS
Mornings	APIS
Motion	ARN
,,	ARS
,,	BELL
,,	GELS

FEELING BETTER BY:	
,,	IGN
,,	PULS*
,,	RHUS*
,,	SULPH
Position, by changing	IGN*
,,	RHUS*
Position, semi-erect	ANT-T
,,	APIS
,,	BELL
Pressure, touch	BRY*
,,	IGN*
,,	MAG-P*
,,	NUX
,,	PULS*
Rest	BELL
,,	BRY*
,,	MERC
,,	NUX*
Rising	ARS*
Rubbing	CANTH*
,,	MAG-P*
,,	PHOS
,,	RHUS
Scratching	PHOS
,,	SULPH
Sitting erect	ANT-T
,,	APIS
,,	BELL
Sleep	MERC
,,	NUX*
,,	PHOS
Standing erect	ARS
,,	BELL
Stimulants	GELS

FEELING BETTER BY:	
Stretching limbs	RHUS
Summer, during	CALC-P
Sweating	ACON
,,	ARS
,,	CHAM*
,,	RHUS
Uncovering	APIS
Urinating	GELS*
,,	IGN
Warmth, heat	ARS*
,,	BELL
,,	BRY
,,	HEP*
,,	IGN
,,	MAG-P*
,,	NUX*
,,	RHUS
Warmth, application of	ARS
,,	BRY
,,	MAG-P*
,,	RHUS
Warmth, of head	BELL
,,	HEP*
Water, cold	BRY
,,	PHOS
Weather, damp, wet	HEP*
,,	NUX
Weather, dry, warm	CALC-P*
,,	RHUS
,,	SULPH*

II

PROFILES OF
THE VARIOUS
REMEDIES

Following are profiles of the various remedies generally included in your household kit.

While most such listings focus on the "physical" symptoms, I have chosen instead to center my attention on the "mental characteristics" of each remedy.

Always remember that when you are in doubt as to which of two or more remedies may be correct for a particular "physical" problem, choose that remedy which best matches your mental state at the time of illness.

This remedy is always the correct one.

ACONITUM NAPELLUS

Common Name: Monkshood, Wolfsbane
Abbreviation: ACON

Description: A tall, perennial plant of the family *Ranunculaceae,* two to six feet in height, with bluish-violet flowers shaped like a monk's cowl—hence its name. It is commonly found in wet, hilly, mountainous areas. It contains the alkaloid, aconitine. The mother tincture from which homeopathic remedies are made is prepared from the whole plant and root gathered at the beginning of its flowering.

Key Characteristic Symptoms: Solid, unreasoning FEAR. FEAR of darkness. FEAR of death. FEAR of bed. FEAR of ghosts. Curative for any ailments originating from FRIGHT. For ACUTE and MOST DISTRESSING conditions. (Should never be given when patient is CALM.) Mental uneasiness or worry accompanying a most trifling ailment. Mostly needed by strong, robust people who have become AFRAID. SCREAMS with PAIN. GREAT DISTRESS in heart and chest. Great FEVER remedy. VEXATION about TRIFLES. INTOLERABLE PAINS. Feels like NEEDLES PRICKING.

ALLIUM CEPA

Common Name: Cepa, Onion,
Common Red Onion
Abbreviation: ALL-C

Description: Like *Veratrum album*, a member of the *Liliaceae* family. A native of Western Asia, it has been cultivated throughout Europe. The mother tincture is prepared from the whole fresh plant gathered in July or August.

Key Characteristics Symptoms: VERY MELANCHOLIC with congestion. VERY CONFUSED with RUNNY NOSE. VERTIGO (dizziness) on getting up. HEADACHE with runny nose. PAIN in forehead. SNEEZING with increasing frequency. BURNING EYES. HEAD feels BOUND UP. CROWN OF HEAD feels SWOLLEN. Feels like eyes were stitched with NEEDLES.

155

ANTIMONIUM TARTICUUM

Common Name: Potash, Tartar Emetic
Abbreviation: ANT-T

Description: Antimony potassium tartarate or tartar emetic is encountered in the form of a white powder or transparent colorless crystals which become opaque by efflorescence; soluble in boiling water and practically insoluble in alcohol.

Key Characteristic Symptoms: Great SLEEPINESS or great SLEEPLESSNESS. Angry DELIRIUM. Sparks before eyes. Does not want to be touched. Thirstlessness. Breathing, expectorating, and lying down almost impossible. DESPONDENT about recovery. HOPELESS towards evening. FEAR of being alone. NOISE is intolerable. ANXIETY increasing with NAUSEA.

APIS MELLIFICA

Common Name: Honey Bee
Abbreviation: APIS

Description: Homeopathic Apis is prepared from the common hive bee. Live bees are placed in a bottle which is shaken to irritate them, after which alcohol is added. After ten days, during which time the bottle is shaken daily, the tincture is poured off.

Key Characteristic Symptoms: DEPRESSED with constant weeping. IRRITABLE, GLOOMY, and INDIFFERENT. THIRST-LESSNESS, ANXIETY, FEAR OF DEATH. Retention of urine. Shrill, PIERCING SCREAMS while sleeping or waking. Redness and swelling. SAD. TEARFUL. JOYLESS. Feels WORSE from being touched anywhere—even one's hair. Cannot tolerate being in a closed room. IMAGINES strange person in bed with him/her. AWAKES FRIGHTENED from sleep. FEELING that the head is too full. FEELING like stick was stuck through head from left to right. Thinks that brain is TIRED and has gone to sleep. AWKWARD and breaks everything. INABILITY to concentrate. IMAGINES that skin is drawn over eyes.

ARNICA MONTANA

Common Name: Leopard's Bane, Mountain Tobacco
Abbreviation: ARN

Description: A perennial herb from the family *Compositae* which is found growing in moist, cool meadows and mountains of Europe and somewhat sparsely in the Northwest United States. Generally the plant is ten to twelve inches high with dull green involucre, purplish hairy points, and tubular corolla with five spreading teeth. The disc-like flowers are yellow and profuse. The whole fresh plant or roots alone are used to make the tincture.

Key Characteristic Symptoms: FEELS as if entire body was BRUISED. Should be given whenever an ACCIDENT has occurred—no matter what kind! After a FALL. SHOCK. SPRAINS. FRACTURES. CONCUSSIONS. FORGETFULNESS. ABSENTMINDED. FEAR of being touched. FEELS as if bed is hard. "First aid" for CEREBRAL HEMORRHAGE while waiting for physician. PAIN as if head was being distended from within outwards. Mental and physical EXHAUSTION. Says there is nothing the matter with him/her. DIZZY when eyes are closed. HEAD feels too large. BEFORE, DURING, AFTER any SURGICAL PROCEDURE. Great for DENTAL HEALING. MYALGIA of any kind. INSECT STINGS—especially bees or wasps. HYPOCHONDRIACAL. NEEDS TO KNOW everything better than anyone else.

ARSENICUM ALBUM

Common Name: Arsenic Trioxide
Abbreviation: ARS

Description: Arsenic trioxide is found as large, vitreous amorphous masses that in time become opaque, crystalline, porcelain-like. Arsenic, an element found in nature, is extracted from its ore and made into a mother tincture by addition of water and alcohol.

Key Characteristic Symptoms: Unable to find PEACE or REST anywhere in bed—continually CHANGES POSITION.

Complete EXHAUSTION. Great ASTHMA remedy. ANGUISH. PTOMAINE poisoning. OVERSENSITIVE to smell and touch. BURNING PAINS. EATS and DRINKS more than is needed. FACE expresses mental agony. SEES ghosts—both day and night. FEARS killing someone with knife. IMAGINES house being robbed. Great SCRUPLES of CONSCIENCE—afraid of offending everybody. SELF-REPROACH. CRITICAL of everybody. LOVE OF DIRTY JOKES. MADNESS due to overindulgence of wine. TREMBLINGS. DEPRESSION and APATHY towards life. Dislike of FRUIT. FURY with desire to run away.

BELLADONNA

Common Name: Deadly Nightshade
Abbreviation: BELL

Description: The *Atropa Belladonna* plant is a bushy perennial of the family *Solanaceae* whose flowers are dull red to purple in color. The flowers are single, bell-shaped, and five-lobed. When bruised the plant gives off a rather foul odor and leaves a dark purplish stain. Homeopathic tinctures are prepared from the whole plant when it begins to flower.

Key Characteristic Symptoms: VIOLENCE and SUDDENNESS. MANIA. BRIGHT RED FACE. "First aid" for ACUTE APPENDICITIS while waiting for physician. ACUTE middle ear attacks. HYPERSENSITIVITY to light, noise, and motion. PAINS that suddenly come and suddenly go. HEAT. REDNESS. INTENSE BURNING. SPASMS. CHILDREN who bite others. DILATED PUPILS. MENTAL DERANGEMENT from ALCOHOLISM. MELANCHOLY after LOVE LOST. SWAYS from one side to the other. APATHY—nothing excites him/her. Desire for SOLITUDE. Great FURY and ANGER. Fantasizes being carried off by the devil or being arrested by police. Uncontrollable IMPULSES. IMAGINES that objects seen are ROTATING, MOVING IN CIRCLES or are CROOKED. THINKS that something under the bed is making noise.

BRYONIA ALBA

Common Name: Wild Hops
Abbreviation: BRY

Description: A perennial climbing vine of the family *Cucurbitaceae*, it often grows wild in the vineyards and woods of Europe. In the United States it is cultivated. In appearance, its root is long, branched, and spindle-shaped, and has a rather unpalatable taste and unpleasant odor which disappears once it is dried. Its flowers are small and greenish-yellow with the berries black and globular. Homeopathic tinctures are prepared from the fresh root before flowering.

Key Characteristic Symptoms: ANY MOTION whatsoever DISTURBS. STICKING PAINS. "First aid" for threatened PNEU-MONIA. ANXIETY. Continually talks about BUSINESS. MO-ROSE—everything causes bad humor. DISTURBING DREAMS. WRIST- JOINT PAIN. Great FEAR of the FUTURE. IMAGINES that everything would fall out of head when stooping. FEELS that head will break into pieces when he/she coughs. SEES stripes when eyes are CLOSED.

CALCAREA PHOSPHORICA

Common Name: Calcium Phosphate
Abbreviation: CALC-P

Description: One of Dr. Schussler's famed 12 Tissue Salts, Calc Phos is prepared by dropping diluted phosphoric acid into limewater. As a compound in nature, Calc Phos is absolutely essential to proper growth and nutrition of the body. It is found naturally in blood plasma and corpuscles, saliva, gastric juices, bones, connective tissue, teeth, milk, etc.

Key Characteristic Symptoms: Delayed PHYSICAL DEVEL-OPMENT of children. DISSATISFACTION wherever he/she is. CRAVES salted or smoked food. Cannot WAKE UP in early morning. FEELS WORSE when weather changes. Desire to be ALONE. Feels complaints WHEN THINKING ABOUT THEM. When BONES fail to knit. Easily CRIES. Grieves and laments over PAST offenses. FEAR of ghosts. FEAR of illness. HOPELESSNESS—believes he/she can never be cured. LACK of will power. MAKES MISTAKES while writing. FATIGUE from mental or schoolwork.

CANTHARIS

Common Name: Spanish Fly, Oil Beetle, Blister Beetle
Abbreviation: CANTH

Description: The tincture of *Cantharis*, a bronze-green beetle with a strong unsavory odor, is prepared homeopathically from a solution made by immersing the whole insect in alcohol. As the creature is somewhat small, it takes about 13,000 dried insects to produce one kilogram.

Key Characteristic Symptoms: BURNING. INFLAMATION. "First aid" for BURNS. FURIOUS DELIRIUM. RAGE. "First aid" for gnat bites. AMOROUS FRENZY. Increased SEXUAL DESIRE. Morning DEPRESSION. Very FORGETFUL. Easily IRRITATED by offenses. Extreme PASSION and ANGER.

CARBO VEGETABILIS

Common Name: Vegetable Charcoal, Black Charcoal
Abbreviation: CARB-V

Description: This is the residue from the controlled burning of beech or birch wood which results in an amorphous black carbon with traces of mineral salts.

Key Characteristic Symptoms: SLUGGISHNESS. LAZINESS. SLOW TO THINK. STUPID. CLUMSY. VITAL FORCE NEARLY EXHAUSTED. Great FLATULENCE. When an ILLNESS was caused by a PREVIOUS SICKNESS or ACCIDENT. INDIFFERENCE to everything heard. ASTHMA. ANXIETY accompanied by SHUDDERING. HOPELESSNESS with tears. Nightly FEAR of GHOSTS. Short-term MEMORY weak—sudden loss. Ineptitude for PUBLIC SPEAKING. INDIGESTION from fats, cakes, pastries. Great IRRITABILITY. CONFUSION in the head. DIZZINESS after waking from sleep. Very PEEVISH. APATHY. FEELS as if hair on head is moving. IMAGINES hot pressure on head. IMAGINES tight strap or handkerchief across forehead.

CHAMOMILLA

Common Name: German Chamomile, Ground Apple, White Plant
Abbreviation: CHAN

Description: An annual of the family *Compositae*, *Chamomilla* is often found growing in temperate regions of Europe. Its ray-like flowers are white, and its disc flower yellow, with the entire bloom measuring about half an inch wide. The plant itself is one to two feet high and contains numerous branches. Homeopathic tinctures are prepared from the whole plant when in bloom.

Key Characteristic Symptoms: CANNOT BEAR IT—other people, himself, pain! Wants things and then when gets them, hurls them away. BAD EFFECTS of BAD TEMPER. INTOLERABLE PAIN. Power of COMPREHENSION DIMINISHED. Averse to TALKING. Easily ANGERED. SLEEPLESSNESS. Feeling as if he/she had NO FEET. BAD MOODS. UNDECIDED. METICULOUS. CAPRICIOUS. "First aid " after a FRIGHT. FEELS as if fingers are pressing on forehead.

FERRUM PHOSPHORICUM

Common Name: Phosphate of Iron
Abbreviation: FER-P

Description: Yet another of Schussler's Tissue Salts, Ferr Phos is prepared by mixing sodium phosphate with sulphate of iron in certain proportions. The resulting precipitate is filtered, washed, and dried, and rubbed to a powder which is bluish-gray from exposure to the air. Iron is found in the hemoglobin or coloring matter of the red blood corpuscles.

Key Characteristic Symptoms: INDIFFERENCE to ordinary matters. Lack of COURAGE and HOPE. Annoyed by TRIFLES. Very TALKATIVE. Unable to find RIGHT WORDS.

GELSEMIUM

Common Name: Yellow Jasmine, Carolina Jasmine
Abbreviation: GELS

Description: Characterized by yellow, bell-like flowers, this plant is a native of North America. The homeopathic tincture is prepared from the fresh root.

Key Characteristic Symptoms: STAGE FRIGHT—FEAR of public speaking, performing. SLUGGISH MIND. EFFECTS of anger, grief, bad news. TREMOR. FEAR of FALLING. Excruciating HEADACHE. NERVOUS, SUDDEN HEADACHE. EXAM FUNK. Great PARALYSER. Incapacity to THINK. DROOPING of eyelids. DOUBLE or BLURRED VISION. Smokey mist before eyes. Rapid pulse—worse from SMOKING. DIARRHEA when excited. FATIGUE of lower limbs after SLIGHT EXERCISE. IMAGINES that he/she sees snakes. SEES black specks before eyes. THINKS that eyes are turning in the HEAD. SEES cloud over outer half of left eye.

HEPAR SULPHURIS

Common Name: Calcium Sulphide
Abbreviation: HEP

Description: *Hepar sulphuris calcareum* is an impure calcium sulphide compound originally prepared by Hahnemann, the discoverer of homeopathy. Traditionally, it is made by heating finely powdered oyster shell, combined with sublimed sulfur in a closed, hermetically sealed crucible.

Key Characteristic Symptoms: SADNESS and ANXIETY for the future. EXTREME AGONY in the evening. Desire to quit work for FEAR of DISGRACE. FEAR for RELATIVE'S HEALTH. HYPOCHONDRIA. General DISGUST. Least thing makes him ANGRY.

HASTY SPEECH which often offends. AFRAID of not being CURED. Always DISPLEASED. DREAMS of fire. POOR MEMORY—especially at work. IMAGINES seeing ghost of a deceased person in morning after waking. Also that neighbor's house is on FIRE. INSISTS on being COVERED even in a warm room. FEAR he/she would murder someone. IMAGINES that a PLUG is being driven into his/her occiput and temples. FEELS like an abcess is forming in head. IMAGINES that veil is hanging down over EYES.

HYPERICUM PERFORATUM

Common Name: St. John's Wort
Abbreviation: HYPER

Description: An erect, branched perennial with golden- yellow flowers distinguished by minute black spots on the petals, St. John's Wort is a member of the *Hypericaceae* family. It flourishes in woods, thickets, grassy banks and gardens. The tincture is prepared from the whole, fresh plant.

Key Characteristic Symptoms: "First aid" for crushed hands, feet, etc., and INJURED NERVES. Alleviates PAIN. LACERATED WOUNDS. HEADACHE after a FALL. EFFECTS of NERVOUS SHOCK. PUNCTURE WOUNDS—from stepping on nails, pins, sharp stones, etc. MENTAL EXCITEMENT after drinking tea. EROTIC thoughts. WEAK MEMORY. GREAT DEPRESSION—inclined to WEEP. GREAT ANXIETY about being dropped when being lifted high in the air. IMAGINES that he/she is suspended in air and not in bed. FEELS that something is alive in the brain. FOREHEAD feels strained. IMAGINES icy cold hand touching forehead.

IGNATIA

Common Name: St. Ignatius Bean
Abbreviation: IGN

Description: *Ignatia* is a small tree or shrub in the family *Loganiaceae*. Homeopathic tinctures are prepared from the beanlike seed contained in the pear-like fruit.

Key Characteristic Symptoms: MENTAL STRESS or STRAIN caused by SHOCK, GRIEF, BEREAVEMENT, DISAPPOINTMENT. SUDDEN ATTACKS. ACUTE DISEASE. "Remedy of Paradoxes." "Silent Grieving." CHANGEABLE MOOD. TWITCHINGS all over body. Behavior is full of contradictions. IMAGINES that one is being SWUNG back and forth. FEELS as if nail was driven into head over nose. EYESIGHT dim as if tears were in eyes. HYSTERICAL STOMACH. Sighs. Yawns. CANNOT tolerate the odor of TOBACCO SMOKE. AUDACITY. Easily FRIGHTENED. FICKLE. IMPATIENT. Incredible CHANGES of MOOD. "Whispering voice"—cannot speak loudly. "First aid" for rectal symptoms. SLEEPS so lightly that everything is heard. DREAMS all night of the same subject. SNORING. DESPAIRS OF BEING CURED. THINKS everything's lost. MISTAKES in writing or speaking due to ANXIETY. Very DELICATE, SOFT, SENSITIVE.

IPECAC

Common Name: Ipecac Root, Brazil Root
Abbreviation: IP

Description: A somewhat shrubby perennial in the family *Rubiaceae*, *Ipecac* is native to Brazil and other parts of South America, India, and Malaysia where it is found in hot, moist forests. In appearance the plant has very small white flowers, blackish green leaves, and twisting, spreading roots from which the tincture is prepared.

Key Characteristic Symptoms: SULKY HUMOR—despises everything. EXTREME IMPATIENCE. Ailments caused by VEXATION and QUIET DISPLEASURE. AVERSE to ALL FOOD. PAIN in all bones as if BRUISED. "First aid" for ASTHMA, NAUSEA, and UTERINE HEMORRHAGES. CONSTANT DESIRE but unable to VOMIT. DYSENTERY. Malaise with SHUDDERING. Tendency to become ANGRY and then to become SORRY. FEELS that head is being crushed.

LEDUM PALUSTRE

Common Name: Marsh Tea, Wild Rosemary
Abbreviation: LED

Description: This densely branched evergreen, a member of the *Ericaceae* family, is a shrub with a very strong aromatic odor. It thrives in boggy ground. The homeopathic tincture is prepared from the whole fresh plant.

Key Characteristic Symptoms: DISCONTENTED with persons all day long. NOISE in the ears like bell ringing or wind storm. CROSS. SURLY. FRETFUL. MOROSE. RESTLESS DREAMS—sometimes in one place; sometimes in another. FEELS WORSE than he is. Cannot tolerate covering the HEAD in any way whatsoever. THINKS that something is gnawing in the occiput, temples, and ears. SEES black points floating before eyes. FEELING that eyes are being forced out of head. DIZZINESS IN OPEN AIR—head falls backward. SPRAINS—especially ankles and feet. "First aid" for PUNCTURE WOUNDS. Relieved by cold. STIFFNESS of all the joints. GOUT.

MAGNESIA PHOSPHORICA

Common Name: Magnesium Phosphate
Abbreviation: MAG-P

Description: Mag Phos, yet another Schussler Tissue Salt, is made homeopathically by mixing phosphate of soda with sulphate of magnesia. The resulting crystals are six-sided, needle-like; in nature, the compound is found in the grains of cereals and in large quantity in beer. It is an important constituent of muscles, nerves, bone, brain, the spine, sperm, teeth, and blood corpuscles.

Key Characteristic Symptoms: FORGETFUL, DULLNESS and INABILITY to THINK CLEARLY. COMPLAINS all the time about the PAIN, for which he/she WEEPS and SOBS. Talks to him/herself constantly or SITS STILL in moody silence. CARRIES things from place to place. MENSTRUAL CYCLES—painful and irregular. OVARIAN NEURALIGIA—especially right side. PAINS—shooting, stinging, shifting, spasmodic. SEES sparks and colors before eyes. Great EYE FATIGUE. NEURALGIC PAIN—especially behind RIGHT ear. TEETH—severe pain in. "First aid" for TEETHING infants. "First aid" for SPASMS, CRAMPS—better by HOT applications.

MERCURIUS VIVUS

Common Name: Mercury, Quicksilver
Abbreviation: MERC

Description: In homeopathy, two kinds of mercury are employed. The first, elemental mercury, is a silver liquid metal which is found in nature. The second is a powdered impure oxide of mercury which was originally prepared by Hahnemann.

Key Characteristic Symptoms: Continual ANXIETY and RESTLESSNESS. Involuntary WEEPING. FEAR of LOSING REASON or DYING. Hurried and RAPID TALKING. WEAK MEMORY—forgets things. SLOW in answering questions. DRIVEN to take long trips and journeys. SPEECH difficult and stammering. HANDS tremor. ROARING in the ears. FEELS as if head was CONTRACTED by BAND or in a vice. Entire head PAINFUL to touch. UNCOVERS himself at night. VIOLENT OPPOSITION to being TOUCHED. Understands but cannot tolerate jokes. FEELS like there is ice in his/her ear or cold water running from it. IMAGINES feathers coming out of the corners of the eyes. REFUSES to do what he/she is told—especially children. FOULNESS and OFFENSIVENESS of breath. Profuse NIGHT SWEATS. POOR DIGESTION—from abuse of alcohol.

NUX VOMICA

Common Name: Poison Nut, Quaker Buttons
Abbreviation: NUX

Description: An evergreen tree, native to India and the East Indies belonging to the family *Loganiaceae*, the so-named "poison nut" refers to the seeds of the berry. The Latin word *vomica* has nothing to do with our word "vomit," but rather refers to a cavity, or indentation, in the seed traditionally believed to be

God's fingerprint. Homeopathic tinctures are prepared from the coarsely powdered seeds.

Key Characteristic Symptoms: "TEMPER MEDICINE." IRRITABLE—sensitive to everything. HYPERSENSITIVE to noises, odors, light, etc. Does NOT want to be TOUCHED. Affected greatly by least ailment. SULLEN. FAULT-FINDING. SELF-CENTERED. DISGUST for life—suicidal. ANXIETY followed by SWEATS. APPREHENSIVE—especially in afternoon. DREAMS of cats and cars. FEAR of DEATH. Continually WATCHES THE CLOCK—time seems to move too slowly. FROWNS and CROSSES ARMS. OBSTINATE. OPINIONATED. DISLIKE of mental work. Cannot get over the SMALLEST HURT. TENDENCY TO RUN AWAY. NERVES all on edge. UPSET—especially after meals. LETHARGY after eating. EATS QUICKLY. "First aid" after EXCESSIVE FOOD, ALCOHOL, or ANTIBIOTICS.

PHOSPHORUS

Common Name: Phosphorus
Abbreviation: PHOS

Description: Phosphorus is an essential element appearing in nature and in the physical body. In homeopathy, white phosphorus is used. White phosphorus is a unique, non-radioactive substance, since it gives off light without heat due to its slow process of oxidation. Tinctures are made by saturating the element with alcohol.

Key Characteristic Symptoms: INDIFFERENT. ANXIOUS. FEARFUL. GIDDY. LOVES COMPANY. "BURNINGS" everywhere—mouth, stomach, intestines, palms of hands. DREAMS of fire and sexual encounters. ANXIETY during THUNDERSTORMS, CLIMBING STAIRS. LOVES to be TOUCHED, STROKED, MASSAGED. IMAGINES head is being drenched with water. Very FIDGETY. FEAR of things creeping out of dark corners. "First aid" for BULIMIA. Sensitivity to LIGHT. BAD MOOD during TWILIGHT. SHAMELESSNESS—takes clothes off in front of others. OPPRESSION and TIGHTNESS in CHEST. WOUNDS bleed very much, even if small.

PULSATILLA

Common Name: Wind Flower, Pasqueflower
Abbreviation: PULS

Description: A perennial herb in the family *Ranunculaceae*, the plant consists of pendulous, bell-shaped dark violet to light blue flowers growing three to five inches high. It grows in dry open fields, and is clothed with long, silky hairs. It is named the "wind flower" since its seeds are scattered by the wind, and called the "pasqueflower" since it blooms around Easter. Tinctures are prepared from the whole fresh plant when in bloom.

Key Characteristic Symptoms: Highly EMOTIONAL. CHANGEABLE. IRRITABLE. TIMID. GENTLE. Easily WEEPS. FEAR of GHOSTS, DARK, being ALONE—especially in the evening. DREAD of OPPOSITE SEX. Great extremes of PAIN and PLEASURE. MENTALLY an "April Day." CRAVES cool, open air and moving about. WIDE AWAKE in evening. DREAMS of CATS. SYMPTOMS appear on only "one side" of the body. LEGS feel heavy during the day. KEY REMEDY TO BE USED BY FEMALES—especially young girls. CANNOT DIGEST fats and rich foods. FEAR of being HUMILIATED. DISPOSED to religion and prayer. IMAGINES that the Devil is coming to take her. Easily OFFENDED. Difficulty finding RIGHT WORDS when speaking. SELFISH. Lack of SELF-LOVE. Upset by TRAVEL.

RHUS TOXICODENDRON

Common Name: Poison Ivy
Abbreviation: RHUS

Description: *Rhus toxicendron* is the old, familiar, garden variety poison ivy. The plant has a milky, resinous, acrid juice which poisons the skin on contact. Damp weather and night are conditions during which the poison is most active. Needless to say, preparing the tincture must be done with great care.

Key Characteristic Symptoms: SAD. LISTLESS. EXTREME RESTLESSNESS—must change position continually. FEAR of being poisoned or some great calamity. GREAT ANXIETY at night—must get out of bed. SUICIDAL THOUGHTS. INCLINED to

WEEP without knowing why. DREAMS of being out walking or working. DIFFICULTY collecting ideas and thoughts. STIFF-NESS—especially knees and feet. INTOLERANT of dampness and cold. SYMPTOMS better when at REST. IMAGINES that he/she is alone and all around are dead.

RUTA GRAVEOLENS

Common Name: Rue Bitterwort, Herb of Grace
Abbreviation: RUTA

Description: Found throughout Europe in hilly country, in rocks and old walls, this strong smelling shrub-like perennial has yellow flowers with widely-spaced petals. Tinctures are made from the whole plant with flowers.

Key Characteristic Symptoms: QUARRELSOME. CONTRA-DICTORY. WEARINESS—as if from blow, strain, or fall. Too much READING or TIME AT COMPUTER. OLD INJURIES that haven't healed. LOSS OF POWER—especially in thighs and lower extremities. "First aid" for SPRAINED WRISTS and BACKS. NEURALGIAS of all sorts. SLEEP DISTURBED—frequent waking. DREAMS—vivid and confused. IMAGINES piece of wood was pushed about inside EAR. EYES water in OPEN AIR and in WIND but not indoors. TONGUE CRAMPS making speech difficult.

SPONGIA TOSTA

Common Name: Roasted Sponge
Abbreviation: SPONG

Description: *Spongia tosta* consists of roasted animal skeletons of the genus *Euspongia* from which various debris has been removed. The sponge is roasted, yielding a brown powder from which the mother tincture is prepared. The liquid is amber yellow and is identifiable by character and iodine assay. Given how it is prepared, the principal components are the minerals iodine, bromine, and silica.

Key Characteristic Symptoms: ANXIETY. FEAR. Every EXCITE-MENT increases the tendency to cough. IRRESISTIBLE DESIRE to

SING—followed by disinclination to work. TORMENTED by memory of past, sad event. DISSATISFACTION with what has been accomplished. PERT. WITTY MOOD. "First aid" for dry, barking, croupy COUGH. HOARSENESS. SAD DREAMS. SLEEPINESS in the afternoon.

SULPHUR

Common Name: Sulphur
Abbreviation: SULPH

Description: Sulphur is an element widely distributed in nature and is an essential chemical constituent found in all living tissue for the maintenance of respiration on a cellular level. Used homeopathically, it is a fine yellow, greenish, somewhat gritty powder that is triturated with alcohol.

Key Characteristic Symptoms: VERY FORGETFUL. DELUSIONAL—thinks rags are beautiful things, that he is wealthy. Must be BUSY ALL THE TIME. IRRITABLE. VERY SELFISH. AVERSE TO BUSINESS. FEAR of giving injurious drugs to people and causing their death. DREAMS VIVIDLY—wakes up singing. Can become WIDE AWAKE suddenly. Takes CATNAPS. PHILOSOPHICAL. CRAVES FATS. Overvalues and collects things of no intrinsic value. Tendency to SPECULATE. "First aid" for eliminating coffee, alcohol, and tobacco habit. CHILDREN dread being WASHED. MELANCHOLY. SEES veil, gauze, or fog BEFORE EYES. Drinks much, eats little. DREAMS of being pursued by wild beasts or being bitten by a dog. Entire body ITCHES.

VERATRUM ALBUM

Common Name: White Hellebore
Abbreviation: VERAT-A

Description: A perennial with clusters of white or green-yellow flowers that bloom from June to August, this plant is found growing in the hills, mountains, and fields of most of Europe. The tincture is prepared from the whole, fresh plant.

Key Characteristic Symptoms: PERSISTENT RAGING. DELUSIONS OF GRANDEUR. "Sullen indifference." Aimless wandering from home. "First aid" for SURGICAL SHOCK. Delusions of IMPENDING MISFORTUNE. MANIC with DESIRE to CUT and TEAR THINGS. MANIA alternating with silence and REFUSAL TO TALK. THIRST for coldest drinks, extra ice. RELIGIOUS FRENZY—believes he is a god. IMAGINES cold water is running through veins. PAIN that causes DELIRIUM. IMAGINES that something alive is RISING from stomach to THROAT. FEELS as if HEAVY STONE was tied to FEET and KNEES.

III

FREQUENTLY ASKED QUESTIONS ABOUT HOMEOPATHY

What is homeopathy, anyway?

Homeopathy is a system of energy healing using minute amounts of safe, non-toxic, natural substances derived from the vegetable, animal, and mineral kingdoms, dispensed according to the "Law of Similars"—an age-old principle that recognizes the body's ability to heal itself.

The word "homeopathy" is derived from the Greek, and simply means "like suffering." Hence, a homeopath treats like with like. Who hasn't heard of the idea of using "The hair of the dog that bit you?" Or has not been vaccinated?

When the founder of homeopathy, Christian Samuel Hahnemann (1755-1843) died, there were only about 100 remedies in use. Today's homeopathy has about 2,000 to choose from—using your spiritual, mental, and physical symptoms as a guide. Thus, homeopathy is truly "holistic" in its approach, and, in fact, was the very first holistic therapy to be used and recognized worldwide.

Following the "law of similars," substances which create disease in a healthy person, will in minute amounts cure disease in an ill person. For example, a homeopath will use minute amounts of poison ivy, *Rhus tox*, to help cure poison ivy's effects.

If homeopathy works, why haven't I heard of it?

Homeopathic principles go back to the time of Hippocrates and the ancient Greeks, but it was only 200 years ago that a German linguist and physician, Dr. Samuel Hahnemann, put the principles into practice.

Bothered by the all-too-often accepted habit of using drugs in great excess (sounds familiar, doesn't it?), Hahnemann tested minute amounts of various substances on himself and his students, and demonstrated that the law of similars, discussed by Hippocrates, was indeed a reality.

He began by treating people with these natural substances, and by 1820 homeopathy had spread through all of Europe. In 1900, about 20-25 percent of all doctors in the United States were homeopaths. Chicago was the world center of homeopathy. There were twenty-two homeopathic medical schools and over one hundred homeopathic hospitals.

A few famous people who endorsed homeopathy were William James, Daniel Webster, John D. Rockefeller, Harriet Beecher Stowe, Louisa May Alcott, and William Cullen Bryant.

However, because of various political, economic, and social changes, homeopathy lost its stature in the United States, although it is still practiced widely in Brazil, Mexico, India, Germany, France, and Great Britain.

In France, for instance, there are five homeopathic physicians for each allopathic (regular) physician, and homeopathy is beyond a doubt the system of choice for the entire nation.

Similarly, in the United Kingdom the English Royal Family has personally used and endorsed homeopathy for three generations. Her Majesty, Queen Elizabeth the Queen Mother, is the Royal Patron of the British Homeopathic Association. Her daughter, Queen Elizabeth, is said to never travel without her personal homeopathic first-aid kit (the very same kind this book teaches you how to use) by her side.

Addressing a dinner of the British Medical Association on January 8, 1985, Prince Charles jolted those assembled by saying:

> *"I would suggest that the whole imposing edifice of modern medicine, for all its breathtaking successes, is like the celebrated Tower of Pisa . . . slightly off balance. It is frightening how dependent on drugs we are all becoming, and how easy it is for doctors to prescribe them as the universal panacea for our ills."*

Recent surveys of more than 1,000 British practitioners conducted by the Institute for Complementary Medicine found the number of patients turning to alternative therapies growing at the rate of 15 percent per annum, with a 39 percent increase in those consulting homeopaths.

In 1977 more than 86,000 persons had attended outpatient departments of the six homeopathic hospitals under the U.K. National Health Service. Now, some twenty years later, who can guess at the number receiving homeopathic treatment from both physicians and lay practitioners?

Although in the United States homeopathy has never since repeated the widespread popularity it had at the turn of the century, a surprising report in 1992 noted that some 15 percent of Americans visit alternative therapists for which they pay more out-of-pocket expenses than they do to conventional, primary care givers.

In 1995, this category grew by 19 percent with an estimated 1 percent of the population using homeopathy!

How does a homeopath think about illness?

A homeopath looks at people as people, rather than diseases, and uses remedies that bolster the whole person rather then just treat symptoms.

Hence, to determine the correct remedy or remedies, your homeopath will ask very specific questions about all aspects of your life, as well as the illness patterns of your parents and grandparents.

For instance, if you have the flu your homeopath will need to know the time of day you felt better or worse, your appetite or thirst, your general mood, and how you are sleeping. This is because, unlike orthodox drug treatment, in homeopathy there are 30 to 40 remedies one may think of when you say "I have the flu!"

In other words, you are always treated as a person first . . . and your particular illness, second.

Isn't this really the way you always wanted to be treated? The key to correct homeopathic treatment is the practitioner's knowledge of the various remedies and your ability to relate the specifics of your disease.

Can I benefit from homeopathy?

Absolutely, yes! Homeopathic treatment is for people of all ages. Since it is a system which strengthens your natural immune system, it is useful for those healthy or ill, for both prevention and cure.

Since it raises and enhances the immune system, it has recently become the target of great interest in the light of AIDS (Acquired Immune Deficiency Syndrome).

Bottom line, homeopathic remedies always heal quickly, safely, and without troublesome and dangerous side effects and actually taste good! For this reason they are of inestimable value in treating children often frightened by medicine.

How do "remedies" and "drugs" differ?

While any substance may be used homeopathically, remedies for the most part are all derived from natural substances, broken down into minute quantities to stimulate the natural defenses of the body. They do not cover up or stifle a symptom. While chronic disease may take time to correct, **generally patients feel better soon after initial treatment has begun.**

Once the patient's own defenses are properly stimulated, health will begin to return. Hence, homeopathic remedies are perfectly safe to take.

Unlike allopathic drugs—administered with the intent to destroy a specific disease organism, and which may also destroy beneficial bacteria and create harmful side effects—homeopathic remedies neither cover up nor destroy disease by themselves. They simply stimulate the body's reaction to throw off the offender, and never create side effects as they work with rather than against the immune system.

How does homeopathy tie into holistic treatment?

Homeopathic treatment is an essential part of holistic therapy and lifestyle, since it recognizes the important mind, body, and spirit connection.

It is totally compatible with nutritional supplements—both oral and intravenous—chiropractic, acupuncture, exercise, yoga, and other "drugless" modalities.

I understand that many homeopaths tell patients to stop taking their vitamin supplements when they commence homeopathic treatment. Do you agree with this?

I certainly do not! In fact, I have been known to say that if a homeopath tells you to STOP taking your supplements, STOP seeing that homeopath and find another practitioner!

Any homeopath who does this needs to go back and re-read the writings of Hahnemann in regard to diet.

In section 94 of his *Organon Of Medicine*, Hahnemann writes:

> *While taking a case of chronic disease one should carefully examine and weigh the particular conditions of the patient's day-to-day activities, living habits, diet, domestic situation, and so on.* **One should ascertain whether there is anything in them which may cause or sustain the disease and remove it to help the cure.**

In other words, Hahnemann isn't saying NOT to use such things as vitamin and mineral supplements—which are natural products like homeopathic remedies—but rather that it is the duty of the practitioner to determine whether or not these, and anything else in the patient's life, may be detrimental to his/her regaining health!

From my own research and observation of almost two decades, I find no evidence whatsoever to suggest that taking bio-available supplements interferes with the action of any homeopathic remedies. The same thing cannot be said about taking various drugs, however, which *do* interfere with homeopathy and actually increase one's needs for various supplements.

For instance, taking Valium for a prolonged period of time can cause a depletion of vitamin A levels in the body. Similarly, taking birth control pills creates the need for additional B complex vitamins.

Is there any particular brand of vitamins/minerals that you recommend?

Absolutely! Since for vitamins and minerals to be properly assimilated and digested they must be bio-available and manufactured according to the highest standards, I personally recommend supplements manufactured by the Shaklee Corporation and sold by independent Shaklee representatives. For information please refer to the appendix of this work.

Shaklee products have been peer-reviewed in at least 70 published scientific journals including: *Journal of the American Medical Association; American Journal of Clinical Nutrition; The Journal of the American Dietetic Association; The Journal of Nutrition; The Journal of Applied Physiology; Journal of American College of Nutrition; The American Journal of Cardiology*; and *Physician's Sports Medicine.*

Exactly how are most homeopathic remedies manufactured?

Most remedies are manufactured through the processes of mother tinctures, trituration, succussion, and dilution. Mother tinctures are made by maceration, aging, compression, and filtration of various animal, vegetable, or other biologicals through the addition of alcohol and water. Mother tinctures are in liquid form and range in color from clear to dark brown or dark red.

Should the desired medicine appear naturally in an insoluble form, the active ingredient is ground with a neutral substance (usually lactose) using a mortar and pestle. One part of this mixture is then mixed with ten parts of a neutral substance, shaken or succussed, in order to form the first dilution. One part of the final product of this process is then again mixed with ten parts of the same neutral substance, again shaken or succussed, resulting in the second dilution and so on.

Dilutions are found in two series, the decimal series which is expressed in "x" and which is based on dilutions in 10s, and the centesimal series, expressed in "c", which is based on dilutions in 100s. Hence, remedies will appear for sale as 3x, 12x, etc., or 3c, 7c, etc.

A rule of thumb is that the *lower the number* in either series the closer the remedy is to the mother tincture or its essential material form. The *higher the number* in either series, i.e. 1M or LM, the remedy consists of less matter and more energy or spirit which has been liberated by the dilution and succussion process.

An interesting phenomenon occurs when remedies are manufactured beyond the 24x or 12c potency. According to the Italian physicist, Avogadro, there should be no trace of the original atoms or molecules at this point, and yet the "imprint" of the original substance has been found to remain. In the nineteenth century, a major rift occurred in homeopathy because of this, with some physicians suggesting that high potencies were totally useless since they contained "no discernible" substance.

What are the two forms that homeopathic remedies are normally available in?

Remedies are usually sold as tinctures, which may contain 20% or more alcohol, or as tablets which are a mixture of lactose and sucrose.

If one is hypoglycemic, sensitive to alcohol, or in recovery from the disease of alcoholism, remedies in tablet form may be preferable.

There is no difference in the effectiveness of the remedy whether provided in tablet or tincture form, and remedies in either form will keep indefinitely.

Some homeopaths say that one must STOP drinking coffee, alcohol, or using toothpaste while taking remedies. Do you agree with this?

Again, I do not!

While coffee may indeed antidote some remedies, drinking it in moderation will not alter the effectiveness of homeopathic remedies. The same thing is true of an occasional alcoholic drink.

Once again, as Hahnemann suggests, the key is what the use of these substances is actually DOING to your health?

For instance, if you are a woman with cystic breasts, all caffeine in any form should be avoided.

Likewise, someone with hypoglycemia (low blood sugar) is well advised to avoid coffee, as it adversely affects the pancreas and trips the blood sugar. Similarly, someone with hypertension should avoid caffeine as it raises the pulse rate.

When it comes to the use of any of these three, they should simply not be taken at the same time as the remedies are taken.

You can have a cup of coffee and take your remedies a half hour later. Or you can take your remedies FIFTEEN MINUTES AFTER EATING and still brush your teeth with toothpaste when you go to bed!

Exactly HOW should remedies be taken?

All homeopathic remedies should be placed under the tongue and allowed to melt, or be absorbed, if a tincture—which they will do instantly.

Remedies should NOT be taken together, but can be taken one after the other and it makes no difference which remedy is taken first or last.

One may follow with a glass of water if needed.

How often should one take homeopathic remedies?

Homeopathic remedies may be taken from one to three times a day if being used to treat a chronic condition. In the case of an acute condition, remedies may be taken every fifteen minutes to once every hour until relief is experienced. Once the acute condition has been alleviated, remedies may be continued once or twice a day to continue the healing process.

Can one take homeopathic remedies at the same time allopathic drugs are being taken?

Yes, but remedies should be taken at a DIFFER-ENT TIME of day than the allopathic drugs. If homeopathic remedies are being taken as an eventual replacement for allopathic drugs, one should consult with his/her healthcare practitioner as to how to proceed.

Certainly one should NOT cease taking a needed allopathic drug until one is certain that a natural replacement has been found and is correctly working—which can only be ascertained with the help of one's physician of choice.

Can homeopathic remedies be touched?

Yes!

Although many classical homeopaths suggest that touching remedies with one's hands reduces their effectiveness, twenty years' experience would suggest that this is just not true.

One must remember that when Hahnemann laid down his rules for the use of various remedies, he was, for the most part, referring to remedies manufactured by his own hand rather than by professional homeopathic pharmacies, which did not exist at the time.

One can argue that modern manufacturing of remedies has made them much more durable and less likely to be contaminated than in Hahnemann's time.

You just used the word "classical." What is a classical homeopath anyway?

A CLASSICAL HOMEOPATH is one who believes that ONLY A SINGLE REMEDY should ever be given for treatment. This is based on the teachings of Hahnemann that a SINGLE REMEDY could be found that would describe the sum total of all one's disease patterns.

This single remedy Hahnemann called the *simillimum*, Latin for "the most similar."

While I confess to being trained classically, I take issue with the practice of classical homeopathy today.

Why?

To begin with, when Hahnemann died there were only 99 remedies which had been proven. Today there are over 2,000 and the total grows yearly.

Secondly, in Hahnemann's time, disease patterns that were presented were "pure," inasmuch as they were not in any way affected by the use of such things as antibiotics, vaccinations, birth control pills, toxic metals, electro-magnetic fields, contaminated food and water, and other environmental factors—which create a host of symptoms that can NEVER be addressed by a single remedy.

Once again, the key to successful homeopathic treatment is to find the CAUSE of the disease and correct it—whatever its source or sources.

What are compound or combination remedies, and can these be used successfully?

Absolutely.

Compound remedies are exactly what the word means. They are a combination of various single remedies which create a new, single remedy which is MORE than the sum of its parts.

It is my belief that if a combination remedy consists of ten different single remedies, the wisdom of the body will select from the compound that single remedy which will produce a healing effect. Once the remedy so selected is no longer of use, another will be selected from the same compound . . . and so on and so on!

Although I agree that combination remedies are of little use when one is proving the effectiveness of a remedy, I disagree with those who would deny their use simply because they are NOT a *simillimum*.

You have just used the word "proving." What do you mean by this?

Unlike allopathic drugs which are often first tested on animals, homeopathic remedies, since the time of Hahnemann, have always been tested on humans, which is called a "proving" from the German verb *prufen*—to test.

Following the instructions of Hahnemann, healthy persons are given a homeopathic remedy and are then asked to catalogue all the symptoms, both mental and physical, they experience.

The results of such a proving is a "drug picture" which when combined with others makes up the homeopathic *Materia Medica*, an alphabetical list of homeopathic remedies with their sources, associated symptoms, and uses that homeopaths consult when searching for a particular remedy.

IV

SECRETS OF A PRACTICING HOMEOPATH

What follows is a discussion of various underlying conditions that almost two decades of homeopathy have shown are absolutely necessary to address if one is to achieve the return of perfect health.

Unfortunately, it is my experience that many classical homeopaths, and holistic physicians in general, do not pay enough attention to these possible causes of ill health and in so doing do a great disfavor to their clients.

Again, the key to successful homeopathic treatment lies in the recognition and correction of the CAUSE of a particular health problem WHAT-EVER its source or sources may be—mental, physical, or spiritual.

HYPOTHYROIDISM

Although many practitioners routinely perform blood tests to determine whether or not the thyroid is properly functioning, some practitioners, like the late Broda O. Barnes, M.D., suggest that these tests are of little value.

Why? Because they are based on a formula that assigns ranges of function to this organ, rather than taking into consideration one's individual processes—which is really what holistic treatment, and especially homeopathy, is all about!

So, how prevalent is hypothyroidism?

According to Dr. Barnes, 40 percent of the population may suffer from this usually undetectable disease!

How can this possibly be, you argue? The answer lies in the fact that an underactive thyroid does not mean that its possessor has to be overweight.

Secondly, hypothyroidism can be the unsuspecting cause of a veritable host of problems that are commonly misassigned to other causes including, but not limited to, the following:

A housewife who wakes up tired, is sleepy much of the day, and is strangely oversensitive to weather changes.

Anyone who has recurrent headaches.

A woman who, despite trying "everything", fails to conceive.

Children or adults who are constantly prone to various infections, especially respiratory.

Anyone who suffers from constant arthritis pain.

Anyone who suffers from severe mental depression, which often fails to respond to antidepressants or psychotherapy.

Someone who, despite trying everything, just cannot lose weight.

Exerholics who, if they don't work out every day, feel unwell.

Anyone with constant skin, nail or hair disorders—including psoriasis or lupus.

Anyone with hypoglycemia, diabetes, hypertension, anemia, or chronic constipation.

Any woman with menstrual disorders—especially PMS—or who is prone to miscarriage.

Any person who does not heal as quickly as he/she should.

Any person who is under great stress or who has lost a loved one or family member within the past two years.

Children who have difficulty with schoolwork.

People who are prone to cancer or who come from families in which cancer is a major health challenge.

Anyone who travels by airplane constantly.

Anyone who works on the computer constantly.

Why are so many people found with this problem? The answer seems to lie in many different areas.

To begin with, many researchers believe that the widespread use of fluoridation in our water has a definite, detrimental effect on thyroid development. Remember, fluoride is a form of iodine.

Here we are faced with a wonderful tradeoff! Will we have teeth that are free from cavities? Or will we have thyroids that function properly? You make the call! I would vote for the latter.

If you don't want to make the call then get a water filtration system, such as Best Water's RO System II, which will filter out chemicals like fluoride. (See appendix for information.)

A second finding is that if you are born into a family in which one of your parents had a thyroid problem—either hyper (goiter) or hypo—it is likely that you may also have a problem with your thyroid. This is why it is important to know the health patterns experienced by your parents and grandparents.

Generally speaking, one may take on a potential for those health problems from that parent which one "favors" genetically. If, physically speaking, you are more like your mother than your father, look there for a tendency towards particular health challenges.

The tendency towards hypothyroidism is definitely something that runs along family lines, although sometimes it can skip a generation, which means that you will have to look at grandparents' health as well. Remember, too, that hypothyroidism can manifest along psychological lines rather than physical ones. This seems especially true if the patient is particularly thin.

In this case, one would expect the person with hypothyroidism to suffer from recurrent bouts of depression, anxiety, and low self-worth. Life for such a person is one in which every molehill has become a huge mountain over which any passage becomes a study in exhaustion and deep depression.

This, of course, leads me to another observation connected with our mind, body, and spirit connection—namely that hypothyroidism ALWAYS SEEMS TO APPEAR in love-deprived families.

In fact, it is safe to say that I have never found a case of hypothyroidism in which a questioning of its possessor failed to yield a family history in which love deprivation was a daily occurrence. "I love you—but don't touch me." "I love you—but don't talk to me!" And on and on.

Once again—body, mind, and spirit.

Similarly, if one does have a hypothyroid, stress of any kind—especially over a period of time—will worsen the condition. Now here we have to come to an understanding as to what this thing called stress really is.

Bottom line, stress is anything that "stresses us out!" It could be a job, a personal relationship with a loved one or family member, or anything in our life that doesn't seem to be working!

The key word here is the word "seem!" When and if we have a hypothyroid, our perception of life is that the legendary glass of water is "always half empty." This is what hypothyroidism does; which is why it is so very important that we recognize it as a possible underlying cause of illness.

One final comment before I tell you how you can test your own thyroid with a simple "at home" test. Although there is absolutely no proof that flying on a regular basis, or sitting in front of a computer monitor adversely affects thyroid function, anecdotal evidence seems overwhelmingly in favor of such a conclusion—especially if one is under stress and has a hypothyroid to begin with!

There are now available services that will come into your home and office and actually measure the radiation from your computer, monitor, and printer.

There are also various devices available that will block this radiation from being absorbed by your body. One such device, the Radon, looks like a large fountain pen and can be worn both when working on the computer and when flying.

Persons interested in obtaining this device are referred to the appendix at the end of this work.

HOW YOU CAN TEST
YOUR OWN THYROID

Although routine blood tests such as T-3, T-4, and "thyroid uptake" will sometimes detect hypothyroidism, the following simple protocol has stood the test of time:

> Obtain an ordinary thermometer. If you don't already have one, a digital one will do.
>
> Place it within reach of your bed together with a pen or pencil and paper.
>
> First thing upon waking in the morning—and before you go to the bathroom or move about—place this thermometer *under your arm*, not in your mouth.
>
> After ten full minutes by the clock, record the temperature.
>
> Do this for five consecutive days!

If the underarm temperature is, on average, *below* 97.8, your thyroid is "underactive" and needs to be treated!

This test is especially accurate if done *during* the second and third day of the menstrual cycle—if you are a woman and still menstruating.

This test should be done by EVERYONE—even if you already have been told that your thyroid is "underactive" and you are on some kind of thyroid medication!

Why?

Because far too often people are placed on thyroid supplementation by their physicians and "assume" that, as a result, their thyroids are working—when in fact they are not!

Once it is determined that the thyroid is underactive, various options for treatment abound and include nutrition, acupuncture, yoga (the Shoulder Stand done three times daily), homeopathy, color therapy, and chanting the sound "THO" on F-sharp above middle C.

HOMEOPATHIC SOLUTION: The author has had great success with THYROIDINUM-3x and his own combination formulas THYGO and THY PLUS.

In conclusion, the Barnes' test is a simple test that could very well change your life!

THE CANDIDA CONNECTION

Honestly, I must confess to more than just a present flirtation with the candida problem.

Almost every day my telephone rings with an inquiry from someone, usually a woman, who has had long bouts with yeast infections, and has found that the commonly prescribed drug of choice, Nystatin, has failed to produce a cure.

But I am jumping ahead of myself, as many of you reading these words may know little of candida overgrowth and its ability to produce such a wide spectrum of symptoms such as: fatigue, numbness and tingling, joint pains, cold hands and feet, food cravings—especially sugar and yeast foods, menstrual irregularities, chronic cystitis, kidney and bladder infections, cramping and PMS, allergic symptoms and reactions to inhalants, hayfever, chronic sinusitis, hives, earaches, asthma, heartburn, colitis, constipation, distention and bloating, diarrhea, and flatulence.

Besides these obvious physical problems, there are also a host of psychological problems including headaches, lethargy, depression, confusion, hyper-irritability, memory loss, a general lack of sex drive, orientation, and the inability to concentrate.

Given all these strange and sundry symptoms, you can now understand why a "classical" homeopath—not aware of this underlying cause—could spend many, many years seeking the right *simillimum* to correct any or all of these symptoms!

To my knowledge, only hypoglycemia, which like candida went unrecognized by the holistic medical community for decades, produces as wide a group of physical and psychological symptoms.

What, exactly, is *Candida albicans* and why is it suddenly a problem?

As is often the case with something newly discovered, its origin lies in the far distant past. So it is with candida, a single cell fungi, that in one type of childhood oral infection, thrush, was first described by Hippocrates over 2,000 years ago!

According to medical historians, vaginal yeast infection (often called candidiasis) was first described in 1849, fungal infections of the nails in 1904, skin infections in 1907, and chronic mucocutaneous disease in 1909.

But it was not until the early 1940s that an interest in systemic candidasis took place, apparently coming on the heels of the discovery of the so-called antibiotic—a word we have been too quick to forget means "against life!"

In 1947, the first broad-spectrum antibiotic, Aureomycin, became available and was followed by a flood of articles in various medical journals detailing the sudden and unconnected rise of intestinal and vaginal yeast infections.

No one at the time, except one pioneer, C. Orian Truss, M.D., saw the causal connection between the widespread use of antibiotics and the rise of the candida problem.

Once again it was women who were most severely affected.

After a course of antibiotics would come the all-too-familiar vaginal irritation, followed in turn by a bout of cystitis. In time it became almost expected that this was the chain of events destined to follow—"I take antibiotics; I have a yeast infection; I take more antibiotics!"

Obviously this was the way in which antibiotics had to work—but did they?

As more and more antibiotics were prescribed, more and more cases of yeast infections arose because now the natural, God-given balance of necessary fungi had been disturbed by those drugs which were not based on the homeopathic principle *similia similibus curantur*—"let likes be cured by likes," which maintained its integrity.

What was forgotten was what was said in that infamous T.V. commercial of the fifties, that you shouldn't mess with Mother Nature! Indeed, for the homeopath, thrush (an early name for candida appearing in babies) was just another example of the truth of Hahnemann's premise that the natural, healing, vital life force must be allowed to operate without interference.

Given this understanding, it is not surprising that we find in *Kent's Repertory* (Kent, 1849-1916) of the *Homeopathic Materia Medica*, a list of a great many remedies "proved" to correct this overgrowth.

In fact, when I first began to treat candidiasis successfully without drugs, I was more than astounded to learn that many persons had actually taken the drug Nystatin for years and were yet unable to get well, when a course of homeopathic treatment would, for the most part, produce a cure in but a few months!

But besides the use of broad-spectrum antibiotics (which is analagous to using a machine gun to kill flies) the present candida crime epidemic has been compounded by the widely accepted use of oral contraceptives (again, a practice relatively new in medical history), and toxic metal poisoning, usually from aluminum found in cookware, foil, deodorants, and canned beverages.

Recently, there is yet another suggested cause for the candida problem—dental amalgams that have been found to leak mercury which lowers thyroid function and, hence, the immune system.

So you see, it is not unreasonable to expect some physical effect to occur when we have clearly fooled around with Mother Nature! In fact, if anything proves the homeopathic contention that antibiotics should not be used, it is the candida problem.

Without going into the problem of aluminum poisoning, which I hope to discuss in a later context, I will simply state that I have yet to find a case of untreatable candidiasis in which high metals were not present—especially aluminum.

This in my opinion is the missing link.

Once the aluminum is chelated out of the person through the use of homeopathy, a healing will begin to take place. This is because aluminum attacks and lodges in the very same mucous membranes in which candida thrive. In fact, it is my belief that high aluminum levels often precede the candida overgrowth.

How does one know they have a yeast problem to begin with?

This is not an easy question to answer. While it is possible to sometimes culture candida from blood, from the mouth, nose, stool, or vagina, or through various skin tests, this may only be suggestive of the possible existence of this problem.

In much the same way, a six- or eight-hour glucose tolerance test may only suggest hypoglycemia, so do various tests for candida often yield a similar grey area conclusion.

Through the use of the Sano Vita Analysis, a non-invasive saliva test developed by the author, candida, and other underlying causes, are quickly spotted. (See appendix for information on obtaining this test.)

Because the use of antibiotics is so very commonplace today, it is my belief that anyone who has ever taken antibiotics should be checked for this problem whether or not they currently have symptoms.

The connection between yeast overgrowth and a tendency towards allergies of all kinds, only hinted at by Truss in his early papers, has been proven in my own experience to be more than just a hypothesis. Simply put: Get rid of the yeast and the allergies disappear. It's that simple!

In fact, it is now safe for me to say that genuine allergies are as scarce as the legendary "hen's teeth."

Ninety-eight to ninety-nine per cent of all allergies are due to either the overgrowth of *Candida albicans*, and other fungi, or the presence in the colon of amoebic entities such as *Giardia lamblia* and *Entamoeba histolytica*—about which more will be said later on.

While yeast overgrowth will produce a host of sinus problems and inhalant allergies, the latter seems to cause a bevy of skin rashes, food allergies, and unbelievable energy loss.

And what about candida and the immune system?

It is here that we enter a difficult ground to say the least. While it is the function of the immune system to keep in balance the presence of *Candida albicans* by promoting the growth of so-called "friendly bacteria," constant use of antibiotics actually tip the delicate bacterial/fungi balance.

Orian Truss, M.D. has suggested that in the case of tetracycline, which is too commonly dispensed for teenage skin complaints that could easily be treated by homeopathy, candida actually thrives on the antibiotic as if it were food!

What has been done to alleviate this discovery is even more absurd, as one leading drug manufacturer now offers a product which, in advance, combines tetracycline, the cause of the yeast overgrowth, with an antifungal drug, amphotericin B! What will they think of next?

This kind of thinking is analogous to a woman going for an abortion the day after she has had unprotected sex on the premise that she may have gotten pregnant the night before! If this is the kind of thing you wish to do to your body—lots of luck!

The answer, dear friends, is not to find another drug that kills the yeast overgrowth, but rather to employ natural alternatives—such as nutrition and homeopathy—which do not destroy the friendly bacteria in the first place! Assuming that candida is suspected, how may it be treated homeopathically?

First, if the presence of high toxic metals is found (or suspected) this must be corrected at the onset of treatment.

HOMEOPATHIC SOLUTION: In the case of aluminum, I recommend and use a homeo-pathic formula consisting of Cuprum-12x, Calc Sulph-12x, and Alumina-70c.

Taken twice a day after meals for five to ten days, this will draw out of the system, without any side effects, any aluminum residue no matter how long it may have been there!

I am always amazed when someone comes to my office and tells me that they have had toxic metals in their bodies "for years." This is absurd, since with homeopathy any toxic metal can be safely and quickly removed, without any side effects and certainly without costly chelation!

Besides getting rid of the aluminum (or any other toxic metal such as mercury), I routinely check for the need for a dose of Nux Vomica—which is used to antidote all the various drugs—alcohol, tobacco, etc. modern mankind is prone to. This is usually taken twice a day for a number of days.

If a person may also have been over-vaccinated, the homeopathic remedies, Thuja or Silicea, may also be administered in the same way as a prelude to treating the candida.

If the person under treatment acknowledges the use of a particular antibiotic, such as penicillin or tetracycline—this may also be dispensed in a high potency homeopathic form to clear any residue of the drug out of the system.

Once this has been done, I now turn to the treatment of the candida itself through diet and very specific homeopathic remedies that are matched to each individual.

HOMEOPATHIC SOLUTION: Generally speaking, I employ two combination homeopathic formulas that I have developed through my own research, CANCLEAR and CAYCE.

Other single remedies that have proven useful are: Borax, Carbo. Veg., Helonias, Kreosotum, Merc. Sol., Sulph. Acid, Caulophyllum, Agaricus Muscarius, Iodum, Sulphur, Thuja, Ant. Tart, Hydrastis, Cadmium Sulph., Ipec., Ars. Album, Capsicum, Kali Chlor., and Nat. Mur.

At the same time these remedies are being taken, one must also seek to raise the immune system, for which I employ yet another formula derived from my own research—IMMUNE PLUS.

Of course, if the thyroid is underfunctioning, this must also be addressed at the same time. While the candida problem is correctly thought of as a problem of an imbalance or overgrowth which must be eliminated in the system, some individuals have both an "infection/overgrowth" as well as an "allergy" to the yeast itself.

These cases are unique inasmuch as once the overgrowth is corrected, a sensitivity to yeast foods and molds may still be present.

This is why one can be pronounced "cured," and still not feel well!

In this instance, one must double back and prepare homeopathic remedies from the offending substances that can be used to desensitize the patient.

While I have seldom failed to cure candida through homeopathy, without drugs such as Nystatin, mention must be made of the necessity of following some sort of yeast-free diet while undergoing treatment.

Although books on candida abound that recommend various spartanlike diets, I usually simply recommend strict avoidance of sugar, bread, beer, wine, mushrooms, and vinegar, together with any foods that may contain these. For instance, vinegar is in mayonnaise, ketchup, and mustard. And sugar is—well, in just about everything!

The key is to begin the habit of reading labels and follow the age-old maxim—"When in doubt, leave it out!"

If one wants to really bite the bullet, the following foods may also be avoided:

Gluten grains including wheat, oats, rye, and barley

Sugar and sweets, including honey and molasses

Milk and milk products, except butter

Commercial breads, rolls, coffee cakes, pastries

All alcoholic beverages—especially beer and wine

Commercial soups, barbecue potato chips, dry roasted nuts

Vinegar and foods containing vinegar—sauer-kraut, relishes, green olives, salad dressing

Soy sauce, cider, and natural root beer

Any meats that have been dried, smoked, or cured—sausages, salami, hot dogs, corned beef, pastrami, bacon, country style cured pork

Dried fruits such as prunes, raisins, dates, figs, peaches, apricots

Cheeses, including cottage cheese, sour cream, buttermilk

Canned juices—especially citrus, grape, and tomato

Mushrooms

You MAY EAT any of the following: fresh fish, chicken, beef, pork, turkey, duck, seafood, eggs, goat, venison, rabbit, frog legs, pheasant, quail, lamb, veal—any meat that is fresh and not dried, smoked, pickled or cured. Rice, potatoes, vegetables—all kinds except those above.

Following the very strict form of the yeast-free diet may very well be an impossible task for many, but it does have its rewards.

Mention must also be made of the fact that taking homeopathic treatment for candida and following the yeast-free diet often results in what is called "die-off" of the yeast!

Die-off, when and if it occurs, can cause a malaise or flu-like symptoms that will persist for a day or two. One can actually control die-off by taking less of the remedy or stopping it for a few days, which will give the body a chance to catch up with the elimination process.

The question frequently arises as to whether or not one should continue taking vitamin and mineral supplements while treating candida. The answer is, of course, yes!

One final comment in regard to treating candida with homeopathy: once again we are faced with a host of symptoms which if treated without the knowledge of the real problem, namely the yeast overgrowth, would simply cause one to go round in circles.

Just as Plato believed that until philosophers are kings and kings are philosophers there would be no end to the ills of mankind, so must the true physician—hopefully homeopathic—become an "informed" healer! But until this happens, each one of us must take full responsibility for our own health. Otherwise we are truly at the mercy of drug companies who spend millions of dollars getting government approval to market drugs that can have deadly side effects. *Caveat emptor*—"Buyer beware" must be our watchword!

HYPOGLYCEMIA . . . LOW BLOOD SUGAR

Not unlike candida, the road to the acceptance of low blood sugar as a "real" health problem has been an uphill battle!

Often disguised as neurosis, alcoholism, lack of sex drive, obesity, exhaustion, anxiety, indecisiveness, allergies, crying spells, insomnia, cold sweats, fainting spells, and forgetfulness, low blood sugar is far too often forgotten as a "cause" of illness despite the pioneering work of the late Carlton Fredericks, Ph.D., Seale Harris, M.D., Stephen Hyland, M.D., and others.

That this should still be the case as we approach the millennium is criminal since statistically the average American consumes about 130 pounds of sugar a year. Imagine piling up 130 of those one-pound sugar bags in your grocery cart!

Surely it does not take a rocket scientist to conclude that any nation that consumes this much sugar is very likely to suffer from some kind of chemical imbalance relating to its consumption!

Is it any wonder that we have a nation of fat cats? That many of us are overweight? The next time you go to the shopping mall, sit down on a bench and just watch people walk by. Or look around at your own family members! Or watch what people order the next time you go to a restaurant! What are we doing to ourselves?

The problem is that, once again, the logical mind part of us fails to connect the fact that our various strange symptoms may actually be due to a single cause—namely poor diet and the consumption of excess carbohydrates. For instance, why should our poor eating be the cause of our insomnia or crying spells?

Another stumbling block to the acceptance of low blood sugar as a disease is the fact that its causation was originally only assumed truly provable through a six or eight-hour grueling blood test: glucose tolerance test (GTT).

This required the candidate to appear in the early A.M., after fasting, and subject himself to the ingestion of a cola-like substance combined with hourly blood draws, the results of which are graphed for future analysis.

In fact, so brutal is this test that one client described herself as emerging after the eight hours feeling much like "Dracula's Daughter!" But the real tragedy of succumbing to such a test—if actually recommended by one's physician of choice—is that one not only leaves somewhat poorer, as the test is costly, but feeling somewhat stupid as well!

Why? Because the *only cure* for hypoglycemia is DIET and NUTRITION!

Hence, it is my humble opinion, after two decades of observation, that if one has many of the symptoms of hypoglycemia, save money, keep your blood, and don't take the GTT—but instead, change your diet and wait for the symptoms to disappear!

In other words, why spend money to be told you have something for which the "only real cure" is a change in one's diet and lifestyle! What the hell! Change the diet, and when the symptoms disappear you can say you *had* hypoglycemia!

So having said this, let's take a look at some of the unusual, and seemingly unconnected, symptoms that hypoglycemia presents—keeping in mind the words of Dr. Harris that "low blood sugar is the diabetes of tomorrow!"

The following list of symptoms was compiled from more than 600 patients treated by Dr. Hyland, and are listed in the order in which they appeared most often in his patients:

Nervousness
Irritability
Exhaustion

Faintness, dizziness, tremor, cold sweats, weak
   spells
Depression
Vertigo, dizziness
Drowsiness
Headaches
Digestive disturbances
Forgetfulness
Insomnia (awakening and inability to return to
   sleep)
Constant worrying, unprovoked anxieties
Mental confusion
Internal trembling
Palpitation of heart, rapid pulse
Muscle pains
Numbness
Unsocial, asocial, antisocial behavior
Indecisiveness
Crying spells
Lack of sex drive (females)
Allergies
Incoordination
Leg cramps
Lack of concentration
Blurred vision
Twitching and jerking of muscles
Itching and crawling sensations on skin
Gasping for breath
Smothering spells
Staggering
Sighing and yawning
Impotence (males)
Unconsciousness
Night terrors, nightmares
Rheumatoid arthritis
Phobias, fears
Neurodermatitis

Suicidal intent
Nervous breakdown
Convulsions

Certainly if hypoglycemia can cause symptoms like this, it is a force to reckon with.

Not unlike hypothyroidism and candida, however, a secondary more serious problem arises when the physician in attendance fails to recognize the hypoglycemic connection and instead assumes that his patient may instead have one of the following conditions—also taken from Dr. Gyland's files:

Mental retardation
Neurosis
"Slightly nervous"
Chronic urticaria (hives)
Neurodermatitis (itching, rash, from "nervous" causes)
Meniere's syndrome (loss of hearing, dizziness associated with it, and noises in the ears)
Cerebral arteriosclerosis
Cephalgia, hemicrania (pain in the head, or in half the head)
Psychoneuroticism
Chronic bronchial asthma
Rheumatoid arthritis
Parkinson's syndrome
Paroxysmal tachycardia (rapid heart beating)
"Imaginary sickness"
Menopause
Alcoholism
Diabetes
Hyperinsulinism (a correct diagnosis but treated with candy bars!)

Unfortunately, the bottom line here remains the same: one cannot treat properly what is not recognized. With homeopathy that aids the normalization of the blood sugar levels, a proper diet consisting of protein and complex carbohydrates and supplements, especially of chromium and B complex vitamins, hypoglycemic symptoms can be totally eliminated!

If they are not dealt with, however, the possibility that low blood sugar will revert to high blood sugar, or diabetes, is highly probable. One important key to the successful management of this problem is something that mothers and grandmothers have often touted—namely, eat a good breakfast and make certain you are wearing clean underwear!

Once again, if one examines their eating patterns they will find that the longest period between meals is usually between dinner and breakfast the next day. This means that by the time the first meal of the day is taken, the blood sugar has had ample time to commence dropping—which it will continue to do throughout the day if left to its own!

This is why it is absolutely essential that a proper breakfast, consisting of a protein, starts the day instead of the usual coffee and bagel or sweet roll. Just as one's car will not function properly if you put the wrong octane fuel into it, so will one's body not be prepared for the usual stress each one of us encounters along life's path.

If you don't have time for a sit-down breakfast, then at least make yourself a protein shake, preferably with soy, such as Shaklee's Energizing Shake. This will at least get your car out of the garage and on to the street! It is of great importance that this first meal be taken ASAP after arising.

If you do not do this, eating a proper lunch will not correct the problem; and this is why many persons with hypoglycemia "die" an hour or so after lunch, often barely able to keep their eyes open!

HOMEOPATHIC SOLUTION: A formula called ACE which I developed from my own research has been found very helpful in normalizing the blood sugar levels. It is a special combination of Jerusalem Artichoke, Chromium, Pexid, and a special form of Adrenal Cortex.

Other homeopathic organ remedies which assist the function of the pancreas are Chamomillia, Lycopodium, Berberis Vulgaris, Fucus, Iris Ver., Formica, Ferr. Mur, Carduus Mar., Bovista, Millifolium, Juglans Reg., Uva Ursi, and Chionanthus.

Finally, some mention must be made of the widespread use of coffee to jump-start our bodies each day. If you have hypoglycemia—or if you think you do—you should immediately stop drinking coffee, which can actually whip the adrenal glands and cause the blood sugar to rise suddenly only to be followed by a severe crash later on.

If you don't have the necessary will power to "just stop" your morning rocket fuel, at least try to replace it with a good water decaffeinated, which, after a week or so, will enable you to gradually cut back and stop altogether.

After you have finally stopped your coffee, a few daily doses of Nux Vomica is always helpful to get whatever remains out of the system.

In conclusion, hypoglycemia is yet another underlying cause that can create a host of symptoms very often misdiagnosed.

If you have any of the above symptoms—and you come from a family in which there is either hypoglycemia, diabetes, or alcoholism, be assured that it's your problem, too, and change your diet and lifestyle to get rid of the problem today before it becomes tomorrow's diabetes!

And don't think of it as a disease but rather a genetic inclination that anyone can overcome by changing their thinking, their eating, and their drinking.

It's that easy!

ADD . . . ATTENTION DEFICIT DISORDER

Have you ever noticed that every few years or so a "new" disease is "discovered" that everyone seems to have? Well, ADD, is certainly nothing new, but the idea of it being a "disease" certainly is!

Just like hypothyroidism, candida, and hypoglycemia, millions of dollars are being spent annually looking for hidden explanations to a phenomenon that is already all too common. As my country Granny used to say when I was looking for something that was actually right in front of my nose, "If it was a snake it would have bit you, boy!"

The reason I have waited to discuss ADD until now is that I really don't believe that most children who are diagnosed with this disorder actually have it! Unfortunately, the number of children who are labeled as hyperactive or learning disabled, and who are far too often placed on the drug Ritalin, has begun to reach epidemic proportions.

Would you be shocked if I told you that more than six million American children now take Ritalin regularly—which is an increase of two and a half times since 1990! And that Ritalin is a Class II drug—defined as a "controlled substance" along with cocaine, methadone, and methamphetamine! In case you missed what I just wrote and what you just read, I said *six million*. That's the number 6 with six zeros after it.

Once again, from the standpoint of natural alternatives, and especially homeopathy, this is truly insane as the side effects from this drug are beyond frightening: such as insomnia, anorexia, hypotension, arrhythmias, Tourette's syndrome, toxic psychosis, seizures, blood dyscrasias, and various and sundry rashes!

Obviously there is either something grossly wrong with our education systems, the American diet, or our medical model that would allow this to happen! Once again, we must return to our basic premise that if the cause of a health problem is known, it can be corrected without drugs through nutrition, supplements and homeopathy!

So let's begin by looking for other explanations as to "how" so many children can be diagnosed as hyperactive, or learning disabled, to begin with.

I already mentioned the fact that the average American consumes about 130 pounds of sugar per year. Doesn't it stand to reason that what with all this sugar around us it is highly likely that many of our children could also be hypoglycemic without their parents knowledge? After all, have you ever seen young children buy candy or other junk food with their own money?

Go back and read the various symptoms appearing under hypoglycemia. Aren't these many of the very same symptoms children diagnosed as hyperactive have?

Symptoms such as restlessness, the inability to concentrate, anxiety, dozing off in class?

Is this a mere coincidence? Or is it remotely possible that a good many of the children diagnosed as hyperactive or learning disabled are really victims of poor nutrition? Based on my experience of almost twenty years, the answer is a resounding, "yes!"

Certainly before I would place one of my own children on a drug as heinous as Ritalin, I would take a detailed look at what they are eating on a daily basis; test for hypothyroidism, which can account for a lack of general vitality and cause depression; test for candida, which can cause spaciness and the inability to concentrate; and also rule out any possible food or inhalant allergies!

Let's start with the daily diet!

How many children—especially teens—go off to school without eating a proper, nutritious breakfast? Do you really think you have to be an adult to have hypoglycemia symptoms?

Over the years I have seen countless teens brought to my office in desperation by parents who will do anything to help their children "make it" in school. In every instance, I have either found hypoglycemia, hypothyroidism, candida—and sometimes intestinal parasites—or a combination of all four!

Of course, Johnny can't concentrate in class. Of course, he has no interest in learning when he can barely get to the school to begin with!

Now, by this I am not suggesting that every single case diagnosed as ADD is a bad call, but that unless these conditions are first ruled out, it is absolutely criminal to simply place the child on Ritalin.

Very honestly, I have seen grades go from C's to A's when hypoglycemia was addressed through homeopathy, a proper breakfast, and taking the right supplements. Again returning to our analogy of the car with the wrong octane fuel placed in it—it just ain't gonna run right!

Similarly, allergies to such things as sugar, artificial colors and flavors, caffeine in sodas, chocolate and coffee, and processed foods with their hidden chemicals and preservatives must be sought out and eliminated—especially if hyperactivity is present.

Frankly, it is far too easy to assume that there is something wrong with a child mentally than for a parent to take responsibility for what he or she may be feeding—or not feeding—his child. The truth is that various children learn differently. Broadly speaking they can be divided into the creative, so-called right brain type, and the logical thinking, left brain type.

The nutritionist, Gemma Gorham, M.P.H., in her very astute educational brochure on ADD (available from Frontrunners—see the appendix) poses a most interesting question when she writes:

> *What if Albert Einstein, Thomas Edison, and Leonardo da Vinci had been placed on Ritalin? We might be working without electricity!*

Again, when it comes to the homeopathic treatment of ADD, the various causes of the symptoms must first be isolated and corrected individually. If, indeed, mental symptoms are in evidence, and are not being caused by other factors, i.e., candida, hypoglycemia, etc., use of the Bach flower remedies has been found extremely efficacious as follows:

CLEMATIS can be used for "daydreamers" and others with short attention spans and anyone else who is always seemingly "out there somewhere!"

GENTIAN or GORSE can be used for those children who become discouraged and give up easily when they don't grasp a lesson.

CHESTNUT BUD can be used for those children who seem to make the same mistakes in their school-work, over and over again.

LARCH can be used for any child who lacks self-confidence.

WHITE CHESTNUT is useful for the child whose head is always filled with persistent, un-wanted thoughts.

STAR OF BETHLEHEM for any child whose schoolwork has gone downhill after a personal shock—such as an accident or death of a family member.

WILD ROSE for that child who lacks motivation and personal initiative.

All these remedies can usually be obtained from local health food stores or from the source listed in the appendix and may be taken separately as needed, or in combination. If I tell you that they will work wonders, it would be a great understatement! You will SEE your child's personality CHANGE right before your eyes!

In conclusion, I remain convinced that the natural approach to the treatment of ADD and hyperactivity in children is far superior to any other approach—especially the use of Ritalin!

Certainly we don't need a nation of children who are being drugged, but rather a nation of children who are drug free! To me, "Just saying 'no' to drugs" includes all drugs that have side effects—not just those obtainable on any street corner!

CHRONIC FATIGUE SYNDROME

Having said what I have concerning ADD, I am not now going to waste your time with a discussion of chronic fatigue syndrome except to say I DON'T BELIEVE IT EXISTS!

Now hear me out before you cut off my head!

I am not denying that there are people walking around with a basket full of symptoms that a particular physician may dub CFS.

I would suggest, however, that CFS is simply an artificial name—an umbrella if you will—given to that person who may happen to have such things as hypothyroidism, chronic candida, hypoglycemia, and intestinal parasites.

It is only when these are all added together that the immune system drops, and such viruses as Epstein-Barr are acquired. In other words, once again, seek out the cause, or causes, of the problem and eliminate them one by one, and the so-called "chronic fatigue" disappears.

Twenty years' experience has convinced me that the search for a "single" virus as the cause of any syndrome is by definition a futile task.

Does Epstein-Barr exist? Of course. But I believe it is a secondary player that is acquired once the integrity of the immune system has been compromised.

HOMEOPATHIC SOLUTION: Epstein-Barr CAN be treated by homeopathy with great success through a "1M" mononucleosis remedy taken twice daily!

You see, as long as we have done nothing to destroy the integrity of the immune system, we can essentially remain healthy.

INTESTINAL PARASITES

If I was writing this fifty years ago, most likely I would have very little to say, since this particular underlying cause was limited to those who may have travelled to a Third World country or who regularly engaged in camping out and drinking from mountain streams!

Today, unfortunately, the so-called Third World harvests our crops, works in the kitchens of some of our best restaurants, and staffs our produce stands in some of our largest cities. We don't need to go to the Third World. The Third World has come to us.

So, too, our once safe artesian wells and municipal reservoirs have become polluted and the task of finding pure, chemical-free water must now be likened to the legendary quest of a medieval alchemist to turn lead into gold!

Just as there were early pioneers who sought to have hypoglycemia declared a "disease," so has there been a few holistic physicians who have dedicated their entire lives to alerting us to these "uninvited guests who frequently come to dinner!"

One such a physician is Louis Parrish, M.D., who has now retired, but who for many years fought a one-man war to get other physicians to recognize this problem.

"Amebiasis and giardiasis are not just tropical diseases. They are here in America, in our national parks and preserves, where the water is polluted by beavers and deer. This serious, unrecognized health problem is compromising the lifestyles of an untold number of Americans," Dr. Parrish wrote in an editorial that appeared in the *New York Times*, August 23, 1987.

In yet another article entitled "The Lilliputian Peril" which appeared in *To Your Health*, March/April 1991, Dr. Parrish elucidates the many symptoms of what he calls "The Protozoal Syndrome," as:

1) GASTROINTESTINAL which can produce oral thrush (candida), indigestion, acid reflux, malabsorption, gas, unpredictable bowel movements ranging from explosive diarrhea to prolonged constipation.

2) FATIGUE: Persistent tiredness, excessive yet unrefreshing sleep, lack of motivation.

3) TOXICITY: A constant feeling of being sick or unwell which can result in a lack of concentration, confused memory, impaired motivation, nightmares, menstrual irregularities, and wide swings in blood sugar levels.

Dr. Parrish goes on to suggest that patients with resistant candidiasis and what he calls the "trash basket diagnoses" of irritable bowel syndrome and chronic fatigue syndrome often have as their basis these very same intestinal parasites, which for the most part, eludes practitioners.

Essentially, when we speak of intestinal parasites, we are referring to two distinct protozoa (one-celled animals) which some of you reading this may remember from your high school biology class, *Giardia lamblia* and *Entamoeba histolytica.*

Giardia is distributed throughout the world in both northern latitudes and the tropics. The infection occurs from exposure to contaminated food, water, or by sexual contact. In the wild, beavers are the natural habitat of this culprit and through defecation contaminate mountain streams throughout the United States giving rise to what has been called, "beaver fever," "back-packers disease," and "wilderness disease."

Giardia is endemic throughout the country with a prevalence estimated at 18 million individuals.

Giardia cysts are shed in human and animal feces, survive in water and are not destroyed by routine chlorination procedures. The cysts are resistant to destruction by stomach acid and can adhere firmly to the walls of the small intestines which makes detection by purged stool analysis—the normal manner of testing—25 percent accurate at best!

Besides beavers, domestic animals are carriers of the problem, but seldom recognized. Because of this particular avenue for acquisition of the disease, parents must be ever vigilant for signs of the problem appearing in their homes.

Giardia is also one of the main causes of "daycare diarrhea," as young children are particularly prone to the disease. In recent years, Scranton, Pennsylvania; Aspen, Colorado; and Pittsfield, Massachusetts have been struck with "known" giardia epidemics. I use the word "known" because I believe that many cities and rural areas have this problem running rampant without being aware of it.

From my experience of almost twenty years, islands such as Hawaii and Key West seem particularly prone to the problem.

Since giardia parasitizes the upper part of the small intestine, maldigestion and malabsorption frequently occur and can produce nausea, vomiting, and fever in "acute" cases, and constipation, fatigue, and weight loss once the problem becomes "chronic."

In some instances, giardia has also been known to produce symptoms of fever, muscle aches, fatigue, and night sweats, which are far too often misdiagnosed as other opportunistic infections.

Given this scenario, then, it should come as no surprise that if this problem is present, even the very best bio-available vitamins and minerals will fail to be absorbed and assimilated!

Again, we need to heed Dr. Parrish's words of wisdom, "I have come to believe that all patients suffering from chronic fatigue should be carefully evaluated for the presence of protozoan infection."

The second commonly overlooked protozoan infection is caused by *Entamoeba histolytica*. Like giardia, this also has worldwide distribution but tends to be more common in the tropics. *Entamoeba histolytica* parasitizes the large intestine and can cause colitis and dysentery. As travel between the U.S. and tropical countries has become more commonplace, so has amebiasis.

Somewhat similar to giardia, chronic, undiagnosed *E. hist.* can cause diarrhea, constipation, abdominal pain, food intolerance, fatigue, and various types of inflammatory or immunological problems—such as Epstein-Barr, fibromyalgia—and may possibly even be a major factor in the development of AIDS.

E. hist. is also endemic throughout the United States with a prevalence estimated at well *over 7 million persons,* though recent clinical evidence suggests this estimate is grossly understated.

Cysts of *E. hist.* are very resistant to desiccation and certain chemicals. They can survive for 36 to 72 hours in 0.5% chlorine solution—which is routinely used in public water supplies. They can survive temperatures up to 50°C (122°F).

Again, according to Dr. Parrish, the medical community rests "shamefully complacent with some alarming misconceptions about these diseases." According to Parrish, these misconceptions fall into the following categories:

First: That these diseases exist only in tropical, unsanitary geographic conditions. It is Parrish's contention that many food handlers in our restaurants in metropolitan areas have what he calls "fecal fingers"—especially food handlers from countries where hand washing is not routine after a bowel evacuation.

Second: These diseases are species specific—passed only from human to human! Nothing could be further from the truth. Besides wild animals that pollute our water supplies, pooper-scoopers, cat litter attendants, as well as bird owners, are all at risk for contracting these pathogens from their household pets!

Third: That an accurate diagnosis can be obtained from a single stool exam. Again, according to Parrish, sometimes three or more samples must be obtained to confirm diagnosis.

(Based on the collective experience of a great many clients, I consider the purged stool test, usually employed, at best only 25 percent accurate. Parrish himself employed a rectal swab technique that together with the use of special microscope stains yielded a very high discovery rate.)

Fourth: That treatment with a single course of an antibiotic like Flagyl (metronidazole) is 90 percent effective. Again, according to Parrish, while 25 years ago this might have worked to destroy this organism, he claims that because the protozoa has now become resistant, today's single course cure rate is less than 5 percent! Furthermore, Parrish found that about 50 percent of his patients so treated experienced side effects to the drug treatment which caused 10 percent to flatly refuse additional treatment!

So there in a nutshell is the picture—and a most grim one it is! But what can be done to change it? To begin with, anyone with any sense whatsoever should immediately obtain a water filtration system which filters out these protozoa.

Highly recommended is the "R.O. (Reverse Osmosis) System II" manufactured by the BestWater Shaklee Corporation. Why? Because it is obvious that no one is safe from this problem and we can no longer rely on the municipality in which we reside to provide "safe water."

Second, all fruits and vegetables that are brought home for consumption must first be washed in a solution that will remove any pesticides and destroy any parasites that may be present. A few drops of Shaklee's "Basic H" in half a sink of water has been found very effective in doing this. (Again, see the appendix for the source for this fine product.) Should this be unavailable, a few splashes of Clorox bleach may also be used, according to some of my vegetarian friends.

Third, great care must be taken that we and our children properly wash our hands after routine bathroom visits—and especially after any contact with household pets.

Fourth, anyone whose health suggests that intestinal parasites might be present should be tested and immediately begin a course of natural treatment to rid themselves of the problem if it is found.

Certainly, while drugs like Flagyl may be employed, intelligent consumers may wish to choose a natural approach instead due to its side effects, which include lowering the immune system!

HOMEOPATHIC SOLUTION: Through homeopathy I have witnessed successful treatment of both *Giardia* and *E. hist.* with THIRD WORLD, a specific formula I developed after many years of research with the health problems of foreign missionaries. Its primary ingredient is synthesized *Lac Homo sapiens*!

Two other homeopathic formulas which work are AM DYS—a combination of Ant. Tart, Emetine, Mercurius, and Silicea and R/51: a combination of Cina, Tenac Vulg., Artem. Vulg., Felix Mas., Merc. Corr., and Graphites.

Unlike the standard drug treatment—which according to Parrish is often unsuccessful anyway—none of the homeopathic formulas mentioned have side effects and do nothing to further the resistance of the protozoa to future treatment.

MENOPAUSE

I don't think that there is a better way to show the difference between allopathic and homeopathic thinking than through a discussion of menopause. As so very much has been written about the subject in recent years, I am not going to bore you with a rote recitation, except to make the following comments: While still in my teens and long before I discovered the holistic way of life, my parents had a good friend who took hormone replacements—long before they were in vogue—and died of ovarian cancer! I have never forgotten Eleanor!

Although the battle continues to rage over whether or not every woman should take hormone replacements upon reaching menopause in order to prevent osteoporosis and other diseases, any intelligent consumer must ultimately examine the options and decide for herself.

Maybe I'm old fashioned, but it seems to me that since, as the street kids say, "God don't make no junk," if He intended women to continue to have elevated levels of various hormones after menopause—this would be happening naturally!

Notice my use of the word "naturally."

Just as our use of antibiotics has created strains of drug resistant bacteria—especially strep—so do I believe that in the future, evidence will appear to prove that our physician's insistence on hormone replacements was a grave error!

But what about the use of hormones to treat the high incidence of osteoporosis? To begin with, it is my personal belief that studies connecting osteoporosis with menopause are greatly flawed since none of them I have seen took into consideration the routine diets of those who were tested.

When the science of nutrition was still in its infancy, many of the early pioneers were quick to recommend that anyone suffering from the symptoms of any form of arthritis should avoid the consumption of animal protein—especially red meat—because high consumption of animal proteins interferes with calcium metabolism!

So what I am suggesting here is that the first step in combating osteoporosis is through nutrition and the discovery of why it is that certain persons fail to properly metabolize calcium.

Remember the Golden Rule of Health: It is NOT what you take into your body but what your body does with what you have consumed that matters.

In another context we have already discussed the work of Dr. Henry G. Beiler, who believed that excess protein consumption, once one has become an adult, is one of the underlying causes of illness. I would suggest that in our great desire to get and be thin we are consuming far too much animal protein—which is taking its toll in the calcium levels in our body.

Second, one of the effects of the presence of intestinal parasites is the lowering of calcium levels throughout the body thereby giving rise to calcium deficiencies—even if supplemental calcium is being taken on a daily basis. So, given this connection, and what has already be said about parasites, any woman who believes herself a genuine candidate for osteoporosis should immediately be tested for parasites before doing anything else!

Third, when it comes to judging who may or may not be a candidate for osteoporosis, a bone density test is an absolute necessity.

But even if such a test shows a definite propensity towards the disease—hormone replacement may not be the best solution.

HOMEOPATHIC SOLUTION: Through the use of homeopathy I have seen great success in the actual improvement of bone density and calcium metabolism by using a combination formula I call "BONE GROW." This consists of Natrum Carbonicum, Silicea, Calcarea Flourica, and Hekla Lava—all in a 9C dilution. Taken three times a day, along with your calcium/magnesium supplements, this formula will work wonders. I remember one client who, after taking this formula for an entire year, went back to her physician and demanded another bone density examination, which he said would be "useless" as he expected little improvement! When the test was completed—which clearly showed a major improvement of ten points in bone density—he still refused to believe the results.

"What have you been doing?" he asked. "I've never seen anything like this!"

"Homeopathy!" she replied.

He shook his head, said nothing, and walked out of the examination room.

So much for enlightenment!

Similarly, when it comes to other symptoms usually accredited to menopause—like hot flashes—once again homeopathy and nutrition offer "complementary" solutions that do not require hormone replacement.

Gemma Gorham, M.P.H., recommends the use of Shaklee's GLA Plus, calcium/magnesium, vitamin E and B complex. Persons desiring to know more about her suggestions will find the source for her educational brochures on this and other areas in the appendix to this work.

Single homeopathic remedies which have been found useful include: Aurum Met., Glonoine, Graphites, Kali Carb., Lachesis, Sepia, Sulphuric Acid, Cenchris Contortrix, Phosphorus, Sulphur Flavus, Platina, Natrum Mur., Agaricus, Thuja, Conium, and Calc. Carb.

HOMEOPATHIC SOLUTION: A COMBINATION FORMULA, "CLIM" containing Aconite, Amyl Nit., Jaborandi (Pilocarpus), Lachesis, Oestrogen (Homeopathic), and Oopherinum I have found corrects most menopausal symptoms. This unusual formula was first developed and tested in India.

Another useful combination formula is that offered by HEEL—a German homeopathic manufacturer—called "Klimakt-Heel" contains Sanguinaria, Sepia, Sulfur, Ignatia, Cedron, Stannum, and Lachesis.

In conclusion, if homeopathy and nutrition can allow a woman to pass through menopause with ease and without the need for replacement hormones why not give it a try?

WEIGHT LOSS

I guess that no work of this kind would be complete without at least some discussion (no matter how brief) of the use of homeopathy for weight loss—and besides I promised the publisher I would at least mention this!

Since the goal of homeopathy is to find the cause of a health challenge and correct it no matter what its source—body, mind, or spirit—obesity is essentially no different than any other problem. As I have already discussed the importance of the thyroid in metabolism, I would suggest that anyone desiring to lose weight should first ascertain if his/her thyroid is functioning as it should.

Second, if one's obesity is due to the fact that one is simply eating more than he/she should—because of various cravings for sweets and other foods—the presence of candida or hypoglycemia must be ruled out. Once candida or hypoglycemia is corrected, cravings for certain foods are usually eliminated and weight loss will commence.

Still another area to be considered is that of allergies. It is often said that one is drawn to eat that to which they are allergic, but what is not realized is that when we do so, there are repercussions in terms of metabolism. On a personal note, a number of years ago I found myself struggling with hypertension for no reason. Deciding to explore the possibility that I might actually be allergic to many of the foods I was eating, I did extensive cytotoxic testing which confirmed my intuition. Eliminating all those foods from my diet to which I tested allergic resulted in the restoration of my blood pressure to normal ranges!

I am also convinced that not only are we affected by various foods we eat continually—even if they are generally considered nutritious—but that the time of day at which we eat may also produce different effects on the metabolism.

I have not yet determined the actual mechanism that causes this to be so, although it is possible that each one of us may obtain a certain "blueprint" for health, at the moment of our birth—which determines not only which foods we should eat but also our nutritional needs in terms of vitamins and minerals.

From my own research, I know for a fact that given certain planetary influences, a person's needs for a particular vitamin or mineral will be increased dramatically, which if not recognized and fulfilled will give rise to the onset of a predictable illness.

One particular case comes to mind of a friend whose needs for vitamin A suddenly sky-rocketed; when not fulfilled, it resulted in the sudden onset of emphysema! In the future I hope to write a book which will explore this idea in greater detail.

Food allergies, I believe, can keep us fat. We can become allergic to any food which is eaten too frequently. Exactly how this can happen is not really known. But that it does happen is generally accepted! In a nutshell, there is really no magic bullet to weight loss other than exercising more and eating less.

The problem is exactly how to determine the "more" and the "less!" Exercise burns calories. If we burn more than we eat, we lose weight. It's just that simple.

Of course, we must also consider the psychological aspects of overeating, if that's our problem. As someone once said, it's often not what we are eating but what's eating us that causes obesity!

Another friend of mine put it this way. "Weight," she said, "should be spelled W-A-I-T!"

Of course, as a general rule most Americans are eating far too much fat and far too much animal protein. I also do not believe—unless you are hypoglycemic—that you absolutely must eat the proverbial "three square meals" a day! In our Western erudition, we have forgotten that in many parts of the world healthy people are found who eat but once a day and usually not from the basic three food groups!

There is no diet that is correct for everyone. Certainly one must consider their occupation and also their genetics. Generally speaking, people will tend to do best when they stick within the food groups their ancestors consumed. If your ancestors were primarily "grain eaters," you will do best doing the same. And don't think that vegetarianism is the right diet for you just because you do not wish to kill animals, or because a guru says you must do this to attain cosmic consciousness! Over the years I have seen far too many disciples already weakened by vegetarian diets come back from Third World countries racked with parasites!

You and you alone know WHAT you should and should not eat!

There are a number of homeopathic remedies, which can be useful in weight loss, including the following: Kali Carb., Hepar Sulph., Graphites, Ferrum Met., Capsicum, and Calc. Carb.

BREAST CYSTS

What with all the controversy over mammography these days—as to the dangers versus the benefits, the subject of breast cysts is often in the news. Would you believe that breast cancer kills two million women each year?

To begin with, I should mention that when it comes to the frequent use of X-rays of any kind—homeopathy has an excellent way in which to deal with its side effects which some experts believe include the inability to absorb calcium in the area so radiated.

HOMEOPATHIC SOLUTION: A homeopathic formula consisting of X-Ray-200C, Graphites-6x and Calc. Phos.-4x taken twice a day for a few days will cause any radiation in the system to dissipate.

I have recommended this formula after dental X-rays, X-rays taken as a result of an accident, for those who fly frequently, and especially for those who spend long hours on the computer—which unfortunately includes many of us these days.

Now, when it comes to treating cystic breasts, even the most conservative physicians are now suggesting that caffeine in any form should be totally eliminated from the diet! This would include coffee, tea, and especially chocolate.

Besides caffeine, any woman who has cystic breasts should immediately be tested for the presence of toxic aluminum in the system. Why? Because a form of aluminum is the major ingredient in almost all "regular" deodorants and moves through the lymphatic system from the underarm to the breasts!

If found, aluminum can be eliminated within a short period of time with a special homeopathic formula already mentioned. In fact, whether toxic aluminum is found or not—any woman with cystic breasts should immediately stop using any deodorants that contain it and replace it with many of the natural products that are available.

HOMEOPATHIC SOLUTION: I have rarely seen either of the following single remedies fail to dissolve breast cysts—Conium-6x or Phytolacca-3x.

What I often suggest is doing a round of one of the remedies for a month or so and then switching to the other until the condition has been corrected. But make sure you get rid of the caffeine and the aluminum!

VACCINATIONS . . . AND WHAT TO DO ABOUT THEM!

The subject of vaccinations could fill an entire book, as it is a subject that has been much debated by homeopaths and others since their inception.

My own feeling is that while they were once necessary, and have done much to eliminate childhood disease, they can cause immunological damage which may result in other childhood illness, such as the infamous inner ear problems that plague many children.

Since vaccinations are often required to get into school, what I did with my own children was to allow them to be vaccinated and then followed it up with a few doses of Thuja-1M, which will antidote any excess toxicity that might arise, and restore the immune system. This is especially important if the child, as an infant, showed any signs of thrush—oral candida—which would suggest that the immune system had been compromised at birth!

THE COMMON COLD

Whenever anyone talks about "curing" the common cold, the usual response is one of great excitement!

Well, I am not going to tell you that through homeopathy the cold can be cured because I don't believe that a cold is something to "be" cured in the first place! Rather I believe that a cold is a natural function of the body to remove excess toxins from the system.

Hence, despite the medical community's insistence to the contrary, I don't believe we "catch" a cold, but rather that we simply "develop it" because of what we have done to our immune system through incorrect thinking, stress, and poor nutrition.

So having said this, I am now going to discuss a number of homeopathic remedies that can be taken to either prevent the manifestation of a cold when its symptoms first appear or how to best deal with its symptoms once it already has a grip on us.

HOMEOPATHIC SOLUTION: For a great many years now, I have recommended the use of a special homeopathic formula I developed called COLD BYE BYE.

Taken at the very first hint of a cold, it will usually get rid of it in short order if taken every 1-2 hours as directed. This combination contains homeopathic dilutions of Virex (a form of Glyoxalide), Magnetic Pol. Arct. (North Pole of the Magnet), and Quillaya Saponaria.

If the cold has already developed, however, or if COLD BYE BYE is not available, the following homeopathic remedies have stood the test of time:

Aconite or **Camphora**: At the very first stages.

Allium Cepa: A lot of sneezing and watering of the eyes.

Arsenicum Album: Sore nostrils and a lot of discharge.

Euphrasia: If accompanied with burning eyes.

Ferrum Phos.: If accompanied by nose bleeding.

Gelsemium: Fast onset with accompanying chills running down the spine.

Hepar Sulph.: Late stages where there is a lot of thick discharge.

Mag. Mur.: Loss of taste and smell.

Natrum Mur: Where one wakes up sneezing.

Nux Vomica: When the cold comes after a day or night of overeating, overdrinking, or a late night out on the town!

Pulsatilla: Discharge that comes and goes, little thirst, and feels better when outdoors.

Rhus Tox.: From getting one's feet wet.

Silicea: Colds that never seem to develop but don't go away either!

Lastly, my maternal Granny on the Irish side of the family (who grew up on a farm) used to be fond of saying, "If you have a cold and go to the doctor, it will take a week to get rid of it. But if you don't go to the doctor, it will take seven days!"

PROSTATE PROBLEMS

Anyone who grows old, soon realizes that along the way various changes take place. First, hopefully we have gotten wiser.

Second, unless we have been blessed with extraordinary genes, glitches appear from time to time which may give us "fits and starts," as Granny would say!

Unfortunately, with men it is often the prostate that kicks up and they find themselves having to get up during the night far too often to urinate. Certainly any man over the age of forty should take advantage of routine prostate screening for elevated PSA in the same way a woman would go for periodic pap smears and gynecological exams.

Statistically, in about 60 per cent of men over age fifty the prostate becomes enlarged (benign prostate hyperplasia) and restricts the flow of urine. Exactly why this happens seems a mystery—except that it doesn't seem to happen to European men as often!

Why? Possibly because for some strange reason, European men often sit on the john—rather than stand—during the first urination of the day which removes the pressure a filled bladder may place on the prostate.

Besides this simple act, it is my belief that just as elevated levels of candida can cause bouts of cystitis in women, undetected candida in men may similarly irritate the prostate.

So once again, if you are a man and have taken rounds of antibiotics, and have not taken Nux Vomica to antidote the side effects from this, you might wish to be checked for candida, and if so, go on a yeast-free program which will assist the prostate as well!

Besides using candida remedies to treat the prostate, the following specific SINGLE REMEDIES have stood the test of time:

ACUTE: Chimaphila-3x or Ferrum Picricum-4c

CHRONIC: Berberis, Clematis Erecta, Populus
    Tremula, Sabal Serrulata, Thlaspi Bursa-
    pastoris—all 3x.

Nutritional supplements which include zinc, essential fatty acids, selenium, high doses of vitamin A as beta carotene, alfalfa, amino acids—especially glycine, alanine, and glutamic acid—together with high fiber diets, rich in pumpkin seeds, have also been found most effective.

SURGERY

Anyone who is undergoing surgery of any kind should be aware of the oft-quoted homeopathic axiom, "Arnica before, during and after surgery!"

HOMEOPATHIC SOLUTION: I have NEVER seen a case in which Arnica-30x or C. was used that didn't speed up the healing process, much

to the amazement of the physicians in attendance.

It's especially great when it comes to cosmetic surgery. What would normally take months to heal happens in weeks! Besides ARNICA, homeopathic CHAMOMILLIA has been found especially useful in dealing with the side effects of any kind of anesthesia.

When it comes to dental surgery, I have also seen amazing results from the use of a lessor known remedy, HEKLA, in low potencies up to 3x. Besides having the ability to normalize calcium in the body, dissolve bone spurs no matter where they may be located, Hekla is a natural substitute for antibiotics when it comes to any kind of dental work.

DEPRESSION

Long before I chose to become a homeopath I was headed in the direction of becoming a Jungian analyst. Having been an analysand of Erlo van Waveren—one of Carl G. Jung's direct disciples—I have always held great interest in the soul, mind, body connection.

While any psychotherapist worth his salt should recognize the signs of clinical depression in any of his/her charges, the decision to treat it with antidepressant drugs carries with it great personal and spiritual responsibility—for these and future lives!

First and foremost, one must always posit the question, "What is the place and meaning of depression in my life?" In other words, I would suggest that, just like any other biofeedback message we receive when we listen to ourselves breathing, depression might actually serve a great purpose—a sort of wake-up call for us to get to work to change those persons, places, and things in our life that no longer serve us!

Viewed in this way, depression is certainly not something that we need to fix—but rather something we need to learn from.

Unfortunately, however, this view does not seem to correspond with that of many therapists and their clients who are looking for a quick fix way to "feel better." To prove this point, it might surprise you that in 1993, Prozac, one of the leading antidepressants, reached $1.2 billion in sales with nearly 1 million prescriptions being written each month!

If this isn't scary enough, how about side effects from this drug which include insomnia, nausea, suppressed appetite, jitteriness, and a loss of libido together with delayed or nonexistent orgasm!

On top of this, far too many users of this "Doctor Feel-Good" prescription have been noted to suddenly explode into psychotic episodes, much to the amazement of their lovers and family members who wrongly assumed that once they were placed on the drug "everything would be fine!"

Given these side effects, does it really make sense to take antidepressants which, in general, are only successful 60-80 percent of the time? Clearly what is happening is that people who do not want to change their "wrong thinking" or "wrong actions," are taking antidepressants so they can continue to self-destruct with a smile on their faces!

Of course, just like children who have been placed on Ritalin so their teacher can have a "good day," millions of Americans have bought into the idea that if Prozac is good, it's good for everything including PMS, bulimia, shyness, low self-esteem, and general anxiety!

When will we realize that the soul of a person with depression is literally crying out for attention? And that stifling this cry with an antidepressant only smothers a message which needs to be heard and responded to? So having said this, are there homeopathic and nutritional alternatives to antidepressant drugs? You bet there are!

To begin with, anyone who suspects that he/she may be depressed should immediately examine the possibility of hypothroidism, candida, and hypoglycemia—any of which can cause depression!

After ruling out these conditions, the following time-tested homeopathic remedies, without side effects, can be taken with great success:

HYPERICUM: Known as St. John's Wort, this remedy, which has been used for 200 years, has just been "discovered," and recently touted as a natural alternative to Prozac! It can be useful in mild depression of the melancholy type.

AURUM MET.: Homeopathic gold in a "1M" potency, taken three times a day, has been found by the author to be an amazing healer, able to snap someone out of a "deep hole" and lift the legendary "black cloud" that often accompanies the need for this remedy—which is for SERIOUS DEPRESSION often accompanied by thoughts of self-destruction.

IGNATIA: This is the remedy of choice when one is depressed—especially from GRIEF, SHOCKS, DISAPPOINTMENT, and full of contradictory behavior, accompanied by sighs, tears, with little desire to communicate.

CALC. CARB.: Obstinacy combined with DE-PRESSION, ANXIETY, and FEARS of all kinds.

NAT. MUR.: DEPRESSION arising from chronic disease. Wants to be alone to cry. Becomes aggravated when anyone attempts consolation. Indecisiveness and lack of confidence are keys to its use.

ANACARDIUM: PROFOUND DEPRESSION. Feels being possessed by "two conflicting wills!" Given to SWEARING. Easily offended. Lack of confidence. STUBBORN with FIXED IDEAS.

LYCOPODIUM: Fear of being ALONE. DE-PRESSED and ANNOYED by little things. Great depression in MORNING or upon WAKING.

LILIUM TIG.: PROFOUND DEPRESSION. Feels like WEEPING CONTINUALLY. FEARS incurable disease. OBSCENE THOUGHTS. Must be busy all the time.

STANNUM: Depression combined with DIS-COURAGEMENT. ANXIETY combined with SADNESS. PROFOUND HOPELESSNESS with FEAR of seeing people.

ARSENICUM ALBUM: Great depression which causes ANGUISH and RESTLESSNESS, and need to move from place to place. Great lack of confidence in any medication. FEAR of death and BEING ALONE.

STAPHYSAGRIA: Violent OUTBURSTS. Great RESENTMENT towards anything said about him/her. Likes SOLITUDE. SADNESS. SEXUAL thoughts.

PULSATILLA: Easily DEPRESSED and DIS-COURAGED. FEARS being alone. CRIES easily in front of others. Highly EMOTIONAL.

PHOSPHORIC ACID: DEPRESSED because of disappointing LOVE LIFE, GRIEF, SHOCK. Great APATHY.

NUX VOMICA: DEPRESSED to the point of not wanting to be TOUCHED. Great FAULT-FINDING in others. MALICIOUS. UGLY.

BACH FLOWER ESSENCES

In addition to the aforementioned traditional remedies, the following Bach flower essences have also been found remarkably successful in treating depression:

MUSTARD: When the cause of depression remains "unknown" but descends like a black cloud.

GENTIAN: When the cause of depression comes from DOUBT.

GORSE/ROCK ROSE: Material and physical DESPAIR.

SWEET CHESTNUT: Feeling of HOPELESS-NESS.

PINE: Great despair from SELF-BLAME.

STAR OF BETHLEHEM: DESPAIR due to some kind of physical or emotional shock.

CHERRY PLUM: PROFOUND DESPERA-

TION to the point of believing one will die or lose his/her mind!

LARCH: DEPRESSION due to lack of confidence.

ELM: DEPRESSION because of feeling inadequate.

OAK: DEPRESSION because of chronic illness.

CRAB APPLE: DEPRESSION because of feeling UNWORTHY or UNCLEAN.

WILLOW: DEPRESSION because of ANGER towards another.

For those who may not be familiar with the Bach remedies (pronounced *batch* as in bachelor), these are a collection of herbal remedies usually dispensed in tincture or liquid form according to the dominant state(s) of the patient.

Discovered by Edward Bach (1880-1936), an English physician and bacteriologist, the so-called "Bach" remedies differ from standard homeopathic remedies in as much as they are not potentized (diluted) in the accepted homeopathic manner. Rather, they are manufactured by floating various flowers (picked at their prime) in spring water until they wilt from exposure to direct sunlight. This essence is then poured off and becomes the mother tincture.

These floral remedies, Bach claimed, alter disharmonies in the emotional states and personality which if left untreated eventually cause physical illness. Hence, by treating negative emotions as they arise, one can actually avoid illness! According to Bach, "So long as our souls and personalities are in harmony, all is joy and peace, happiness and health. It is when our personalities are led astray from the path laid down by the soul, either by our own worldly desires or by the persuasion of others, that a conflict arises. This conflict is the root cause of disease and unhappiness."

Before his transition (death) in 1936, Bach isolated 39 essences, corresponding to various emotional states, which have been used worldwide with great success.

Persons desiring to use the Bach remedies are referred to the appendix for more information regarding these amazing healers.

LYME DISEASE

Every few years or so a particular disease comes to the fore and seemingly overnight becomes the favored topic of coffee clatches and housewives everywhere. Such a disease is Lyme disease which was first named after Old Lyme, the community in Connecticut where it was first diagnosed.

What with the populous deer herd in New England, the mid-Atlantic region, and as far west as Minnesota and Wisconsin, it is not surprising that this disease is caused by a spiral shaped bacteria, *Borrelia burgdorferi*, spread through the bite of the deer tick—which in turn "bites" unsuspecting hikers, campers, and anyone mowing the lawn.

Just as in our previous discussion of intestinal parasites, once again we find the fallacy of presuming a disease to be "species specific." Hence, one has to pose the next logical question: "What happens if the deer tick bites a household pet? Can one then acquire the disease from the pet?"

I would have to assume the answer is a resounding "yes," which may account for the presence of the disease in some persons who have clearly not been bitten! Characterized by a large bull's-eye rash that has a clear center and red circles of inflammation, persons who are bitten develop flu-like symptoms—headache, fever, swollen glands, stiff neck, and painful arthritis-like joints—especially if the tick is not discovered and promptly removed.

In appearance the tick itself is a tiny, dark brown bug with a round body and eight legs.

A major problem in diagnosis is the fact that not everyone who has contracted the disease may recall the "ring-like" rash, especially if it has already spread on to different parts of the body before medical help is obtained or has been assumed to be some kind of allergy and initially ignored!

Sometimes, too, patients may be misdiagnosed as having rheumatoid arthritis. Once Lyme is suspected, however, diagnosis is usually confirmed by special blood tests and followed by excessive rounds of the drug tetracycline, once dispensed like candy for teenage acne.

Does tetracycline have side effects? It does! They include nausea, dizziness, photosensitivity, liver toxicity, increased BUN, GI upsets and its own rash! So given these side effects is there a homeopathic or nutritional treatment for this problem? Absolutely!

In terms of nutrition, mega doses of vitamin C, together with garlic, and other foods rich in vitamin C, have been found to help those diagnosed recover more quickly.

HOMEOPATHIC SOLUTION: The remedy Ledum in a "1M" potency, taken three times a day, has been found highly successful in treating this problem and can also be used prophylactically as well.

A combination of homeopathic colloidal silver, gold, and copper has also been found extremely useful. Lastly, the use of two combination formulas, BLOOD 200 (China, Chinin Sulph., Cuprem Met., Ferrum Met., Nat. Mur., Pancreatin, Phosphoric Acid and Phosphorus), and IMMUNE PLUS (a special formula developed by the late Ruth Drown, D.C.) has been successful in aiding the immune system to deal with the infection.

IMPOTENCY

As these words are being written, more and more stories are hitting the media surrounding the new drug, Viagra, and its potential to fuel the fires of passion for every would-be Casanova.

One statistic claims that between 20 and 30 million men suffer from erectile dysfunction, and that only 5 percent of them are showing up in physicians' offices to seek help.

Yet another statistic would place the number of American men who are consistently unable to maintain erections at 15 million—and 80 to 90 percent of the time, the cause is "physical."

If true, the reticence regarding sexual health

problems would match the experience of psychologists and sex therapists who have long held that most persons just don't talk about such things!

Of course, when it comes to men and the male ego, very few are willing to admit they have a problem—although their unfulfilled lovers and wives would be quick to say otherwise!

While the Victorian Age may have long since gone, remnants of it seem to persist in the bedroom despite the fact that blatant references to sexual performance abound on our television screens, in movies, and in our daily press.

Surely if someone is willing to pay the outrageous price of ten dollars, and upwards, for a single Viagra pill, lack of successful male sexual performance may indeed be the best kept secret since the atom bomb!

Personally, I would take umbrage at the use of the word "physical." Although various experts would surely agree that impotency manifests on the physical plane, I would counter that at least 90 percent of a man's ability to perform is in the "mind"—which in turn affects the body! But there are some interesting physical connections.

One such is the observation of J. D. Wallach, D.V.M., N.D., who notes that bulls placed on low cholesterol diets consistently lose their desire to mate! This is particularly interesting, since low sperm counts have been reported to be on the rise worldwide, providing fuel for a host of problems associated with couples who are unable to conceive.

Along similar lines, any man taking prescription drugs for anything from cholesterol to blood pressure should investigate the proven side effects which far too often include a "loss of libido."

So having said all this, what can we do from a nutritional and homeopathic standpoint?

Nutritionally speaking, levels of vitamins A and E should be examined along with the mineral, zinc.

HOMEOPATHIC SOLUTION: Two combination remedies have been found useful for this problem. The first consists of Calc. Phos.-6x, Kali Phos.-6x, Kali Sulph.-10c, and Nat. Phos.-6x. This should be taken once daily.

Another useful formula consists of Zingiber-3x, Platina-30c, Phos. Acid-6x, Yohimbinum-lx, and Orchitinum-1x. This should also be taken once daily.

SINGLE HOMEOPATHIC remedies include: Agnus Castus, Conium, Sepia, Sulphur, Lycopodium, Graphites, Kali Bich. and Kali Carb.

Remember that a man's sex drive is ultimately a reflection of his mind, body, spirit!

Hence, if anyone is in ill health . . . or depressed . . . sex drive and the inability to perform may be just another symptom of one's dis-ease. Again, the Bach flower remedies may be helpful if one's mental state is a factor.

One thing is certain; before you run out and refinance your home to pay for a year's supply of Viagra, you should certainly try some natural alternatives which have stood the test of time, have no side effects, and WORK!

POSTSCRIPT

Remember that old saw. . . "What goes around comes around?"

We started our discussion with an endorsement of homeopathy as the clear alternative to antibiotics for obvious reasons—not just its absence of side effects.

But now, regretfully, we end our discussion on a more somber note—namely, if we persist in the indiscriminate use of antibiotics, we are very likely to destroy all forms of life as we currently know them!

That this handwriting is already on the wall is evidenced by the following news release from the *New York Post* wire services on August 22, 1997, which I reproduce below in its entirety:

Drug-proof Killer Germ Reaches U.S.

Atlanta—A staph germ that has resisted medicine's drug of last resort has **shown up for the first time in the United States**, the government said yesterday. "The timer is going off," said Dr. William Jarvis, a medical epidemiologist with the Centers for Disease Control and Prevention.

"We were concerned it would emerge here. (Now) it has emerged here, and we are concerned we're going to see it popping up in more places."

Staph bacteria are the number one cause of hospital infections, and kill 60,000 to 80,000 Americans a year.

Penicillin was a wonder drug that killed staph when the drug became available in 1947. But within a decade, some strains of staph grew resistant.

Medicine's latest "silver bullet" to kill staph is vancomycin.

But in July, a strain of *Staphylococcus aureus* bacteria found in a Michigan man showed an intermediate level of resistance to vancomycin—one step from immunity to the drug, the CDC said.

The man, who was not identified, is now being treated with a combination of drugs, including vancomycin, Jarvis said.

The Michigan discovery came three months after a similar resistant strain was found in Japan.

"Now that you have two in such a short time, there will be heightened concern," said Richard Schwalbe, director of clinical microbiology at the University of Maryland.

The bacteria can collect on clothing, blankets, walls and medical equipment. Hospital workers can pass them on by hand, and they can cling to tubes inserted into the body.

To combat the germs' spread, many hospitals across the country have restricted use of their most potent antibiotics and isolated their sickest patients.

Jarvis said the new strain is rare and should not deter people from seeking hospital care.

"The majority of people aren't going to be in danger of getting this," he said.

OMNIA TEMPUS REVELAT!

APPENDIX

Following are sources for information and products mentioned in the foregoing text. When requesting information, please mention you read about their products or services in *Homeopathy Made Simple*.

BACH FLOWER REMEDIES:

Local sources for obtaining the Bach flower remedies together with nationwide training programs on how to use the remedies.

Nelson Bach USA, Ltd.
100 Research Drive
Wilmington, MA 01887
General Information: 800-319-9151
Education: 800-334-0843

BROCHURES & EDUCATIONAL MATERIALS BY GEMMA GORHAM, M.P.H., NUTRITIONIST:

These easy-to-use nutritional brochures and herb panels cover a variety of health concerns such as ADD, menopause, women's health, depression, children's nutrition, candida, hypoglycemia, etc.; include recommendations for specific vitamins, minerals, herbs, diet, etc. Also available on audio- and video-tapes. For complete list write or call:

THE FRONTRUNNERS
1820 Homestead Trail
Long Lake, MN 55356-9352
800-237-5199, Fax 612-475-3715

HOMEOPATHIC BOOKS:

Offers the most comprehensive catalog of homeopathic information available anywhere in the U.S.

Dana Ullman, M.P.H.
Homeopathic Educational Services
2124 Kittredge Street
Berkeley, CA 94704
510-649-0294 (9 a.m.-6 p.m. CPT)
800-359-9051, Fax 510-649-1955

HOMEOPATHY, NUTRITIONAL MEDICINE AND ALLERGIES:

Philip L. Bonnet, M.D., P.C.
1086 Taylorsville Road
Washington Crossing, PA 18977
215-321-8321, Fax 215-321-9837

HOMEOPATHIC HOUSEHOLD KITS:

THE FRONTRUNNERS
1820 Homestead Trail
Long Lake, MN 55356-9352
800-237-5199, Fax 612-475-3715

SHAKLEE SUPPLEMENTS & BEST WATER SYSTEMS:

Check your local Yellow Pages. If you cannot find them, or need additional information call:

877-306-3239
Toll Free: 800-826-1705
800-766-5457

RADIATION AND ELECTRO-MAGNETIC PROTECTION DEVICES:

For information on the Radon, a device that can be worn to prevent absorption of X-rays, etc., and other shielding equipment.

PSITECH
PO Box 461
Fox Lake, IL 60020
800-726-1880
Fax 815-363-7266

For information on other radiation shielding devices, testing meters, etc.

BEFIT ENTERPRISES
PO Box 5034
Southampton, NY 11969
800-497-9516

For information on approved testing devices:

NEFTA
National Electromagnetic Field Testing Assoc.
628-B Library Place
Evanston, IL 60201
847-475-3696

COLOR THERAPY:

The best single source for the latest developments in color therapy and research. Publishes periodic newsletters, various books on color.

DINSHAH HEALTH SOCIETY
100 Dinshah Drive
Malaga, NJ 08328
609-692-4686

SANO VITA ANALYSIS AND VARIOUS HOMEOPATHIC FORMULAS:

For information on the research and teachings of Dr. R. Donald Papon and his various formulas referenced in this work.

PO Box 31
Lambertville, NJ 08530
1-877-869-1704 (toll free)

FURTHER READING

Airola, Dr. Paavo. *Hypoglycemia: A Better Approach.* Sherwood, OR: Health Plus, 1977.

Allen, M.D., Timothy F. *The Encyclopedia of Pure Materia Medica.* New Delhi: B. Jain Publishers, Ltd., 1982.

Anderson, Nina & Peiper, Howard. *A.D.D.: The Natural Approach.* E. Canaan, CT: Safe Goods, 1996.

Bach, M.D., Edward. *THE BACH FLOWER REMEDIES: Heal Thyself, The Twelve Healers, The Bach Remedies Repertory.* New Canaan, CT: Keats Publishing, Inc., 1979.

Barnard, Julian, Editor. *Collected Writings of Edward Bach.* Herford, UK: Bach Educational Programme, 1987.

A Guide to the Bach Flower Remedies. Essex, UK: The C.W. Daniel Company, Ltd., 1979.

Barnes, M.D., Broda O. *HYPO-THYROIDISM: The Unsuspected Illness.* New York: Harper & Row, 1976.

Bieler, M.D., Henry G. *Food Is Your Best Medicine.* New York: Ballantine Books, 1965.

Boericke, M.D., William & Dewey, Willis A. *The Twelve Tissue Remedies of Schussler.* New Delhi: B. Jain Publishers, Ltd., 1982.

Boericke, M.D., William. *Materia Medica with Repertory.* Philadelphia: Boericke & Runyon, 1927.

Chancellor, Dr. Philip M. *Handbook of the Bach Flower Remedies.* London, England: The C.W. Daniel Company, Ltd., 1971.

Clarke, M.D., John Henry. *A Clinical Repertory to the Dictionary of Materia Medica.* N. Devon, UK: Health Science Press, 1979.
———*A Dictionary of the Practical Materia Medica.* New Delhi: B. Jain Publishers, Ltd., 1978.

Cook, Dr. Trevor M. *The A-Z of Homeopathy.* Berkshire, UK: W. Foulsham & Co., Ltd., 1985.

Cummins, F.N.P., Stephen & Dana Ullman, M.P.H. *Everybody's Guide to Homeopathic Remedies.* Los Angeles: Jeremy P. Tarcher, Inc., 1984.

Fredericks, Ph.D., Carlton. *Low Blood Sugar and You.* New York: Charter, 1969.

Gallavardin, Dr. Jean-Pierre. *Repertory of Psychic Medicines with Materia Medica.* New Delhi: B. Jain Publishers, Ltd., 1991.

Hahnemann, Samuel. *Organon of Medicine.* Los Angeles: Jeremy P. Tarcher, Inc., 1982.

Horvilleur, M.D., Alain. *The Family Guide to Homeopathy.* Virginia: Health & Homeopathy Publishing, Inc., 1986.

Howard, Judy & John Ramsell. *The Original Writings of Edward Bach*. Essex, England: The C.W. Daniel Company, Ltd., 1990.

Julian, O.A. *Materia Medica of New Homoeopathic Remedies*. Beaconsfield, UK: Beaconsfield Publishers, Ltd., 1979.

Krishnamoorty, Dr. V. *Beginner's Guide to Bach Flower Remedies, Part I & II*. New Delhi: B. Jain Publishers, Ltd., 1979.

Levy, M.D., Michel M. Bouko. *Homeopathic & Drainage Repertory*. Editions Similia, 1992

Lorenzani, Ph.D., Shirley S. *CANDIDA: A Twentieth Century Disease*. New Canaan CT: Keats Publishing Co., 1986.

Maury, Dr. E.A. *Homeopathic Practice in 30 Remedies*. Wellingborough, UK: Thorsons Publishers, Ltd., 1978.

Patersimilias. *A Song of Symptoms*. N. Devon, UK: Health Science Press, 1974.

Petrak, Joyce. *BACH FLOWER REMEDIES: Humor to Remember Them*. Lenoir City, TN: Curry-Peterson Press, 1991.

Powell, Eric F.W. *Biochemistry Up To Date*. Devon, UK: Health Science Press, 1963.

Roberts, M.D., Herbert A. *Sensations As If*. New Delhi: B. Jain Publishing, 1937

Scheffer, Mechthild. *Bach Flower Therapy—Theory and Practice*. Rochester, VT: Healing Arts Press, 1988.

Shepherd, Dr. Dorothy. *Magic of the Minimum Dose*. N. Devon, UK: Health Science Press, 1964.

———. *More Magic of the Minimum Dose*. N. Devon, UK: Health Science Press, 1974.

Smith, Trevor. *Homeopathic Medicine*. Wellingborough, UK: Thorsons Publishers, Ltd., 1982.

Speight, Phyllis. *A Study Course in Homeopathy*. N. Devon, UK: Health Science Press, 1979.

Stephenson, M.D., James H. *A Doctor's Guide to Helping Yourself with Homeopathic Remedies*. West Nyack, NY: Parker Publishing Co., 1976.

Stoff, M.D., Jesse A. & Pellegrino, Ph.D., Charles R. *CHRONIC FATIGUE SYNDROME: The Hidden Epidemic*. New York: Harper Perennial, 1992.

Truss, M.D., C. Orian. *The Missing Diagnosis*. Birmingham, AL, 1982.

Tyler, M.L. *Homeopathic Drug Pictures*. Devon, UK: Health Science Press, 1952.

Vithoulkas, George. *The Science of Homeopathy*. New York: Grove Press, Inc., 1980.

———. *HOMEOPATHY: Medicine of the New Man*. Wellingborough, UK: Thorsons Publishers Limited, 1979

Weiner, Michael & Goss, Kathleen. *The Complete Book of Homeopathy*. New York: Bantam Books, 1981.

Index

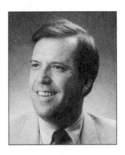

About the Author

R. Donald Papon, B.A., D.Sc., D. Hom., has dedicated much of his adult life to teaching holistic living incorporating mind, body, and spirit. He received his bachelor of arts degree in philosophy from The New School for Social Research in 1961 and then went on to earn graduate degrees in holistic health, nutrition, and his Doctor of Homeopathic Medicine from the Institutum Internationale Homeopathie in Mexico in 1983.

An ordained New Thought minister, he served as associate minister for church growth with the Quimby Memorial Church, and is a frequent speaker at various Unity and Science of Mind churches. He is an analysand of Erlo van Waveren, a direct disciple of Carl Gustav Jung. His original intent was to go to Zurich and become a "Jungian analyst," until dreams from his own therapy led him to homeopathy instead.

He has served as an adjunct lecturer at the New School, Hunter College, and Brooklyn College and as a consulting homeopath, with private practices in New York and Florida, for almost two decades. Dr. Papon has lived in Key West and Princeton, and currently resides in the Victorian seaside town of Ocean Grove, New Jersey, with, in his own words, 'far too many books and ideas!"

Hampton Roads Publishing Company

. . . for the evolving human spirit

Hampton Roads Publishing Company
publishes books on a variety of subjects including
metaphysics, health, complementary medicine,
visionary fiction, and other related topics.

For a copy of our latest catalog,
call toll-free, 800-766-8009,
or send your name and address to:

Hampton Roads Publishing Company, Inc.
134 Burgess Lane
Charlottesville, VA 22902
e-mail: hrpc@hrpub.com
www.hrpub.com